THE 20 PENNIES
A DAY DIET
PLAN

HOW I LOST 100 POUNDS USING
20 PENNIES A DAY!

BY FRANK M. CONAWAY, JR.

ISBN 978-0-578-10079-1

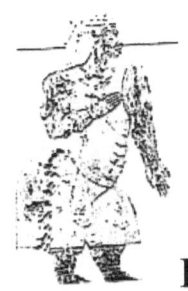

How I Lost One Hundred Pounds:

The 20 Pennies A Day Diet Plan:

A Declaration Of War Against Corpulence

Obesity And The Attack There Of!

By: Frank M. Conaway, Jr.

< Emergency Manuscript Edition One >

TITLE PAGE

"HOW I LOST ONE HUNDRED POUNDS":

THE 2O PENNIES A DAY DIET PLAN:

THE <u>TECHNICAL</u> NAME:

THE LOW CARB < LOW CARBOHYDRATE > LIPOLYSIS KETOSIS HYDRATION THERMAL INTESTINE KETOGENIC DIET PLAN

FRANK M. CONAWAY, JR.

CONTENTS

DEDICATION

REACHING OUT

Dear Friends, I am writing this in a sincere effort to reach the many people whom may have a similar weight problem like I did. To be honest, I was twice the size I am now. I sought help from all available sources, but to not avail. But I never gave up hope and faith. The short of it is this has been a lifetime annoyance. I did at times have certain victories only to fall again. And the pain associated with the weight problem should be called to suffer in silence. I have known the pain, but I don't know which pain was greater; the physical pain of my own body or the mental pain inflicted upon me by some who "said" they cared about me. Near the end of my struggle, I had become a giant. I was a giant because of the sound of breaking concrete under my massive widen feet. Boom, Boom, Boom! And of course, my heart was functioning at peek performance due to the pounding sound I could hear within my chest. And then there were my massive lungs, which I consistently filled to capacity. I sure was sucking up a lot of air. I used to look forward to night time. No, that is not the reason, but so I could lie down but I found out quickly that I could get no rest due to body pains and leg ackes. So I generally was never comfortable. And that terrible walk from the front door to the car door. Oh happy day, as I would slide, fall into the seat. That rocking motion did make me feel better. Then of course if let the car thoroughly warm up, while I caught my breath and those long scenic rides in anticipation of reaching the store. My, you learn and practice patience, looking waiting for a parking spot close to the stores door. Then on day it happened, I saw something awful and decided it was now or never. So I began to combine my research and purify my plan of weight loss. I was fighting for my own life. And so I made some advancement. Then a terrible thing happened to me. The unthinkable. Lets call it vechiluar anger. Suddenly, I was forced to take a short walk to the bus stop in the morning and from it in the evenings. Oh about fifty minutes for a fifteen minute walk. And the burn in my feet and legs, plus a good old dry mouth with the sticky tongue. Each and every block I would give myself the "don't pass out, until the end of this block"! I would argue with myself about the validity of stopping, only to start again and the affects of latic acid. You know, it's nothing like sweating profusely in the darkness of morning. Alright, I will admit it, once I did let the first bus go pass. I was too tired to get on, and it was morning. And then I found out that I was the object of jokes by a certain group of people. It was as if the wanted to see me suffer. So, suffer I did. I decreased my walking time by focusing blocks ahead and crying as freely as wanted. But I said: "One Day!" Results were slow, but I continued to purify my system. Then I had a certain so called supposed to be friend ask me to help the mow their lawn. Alright, I'll try. Well, a gas powered push mower. Oh, about three rows and then I stopped. "Look, why don't you just pay somebody" to my face. "Why don't your lazy fat etc!" Needless to say, that particular friend's anger and attitude has not gotten any better even unto today. Critic! I can truly say that it was the worst year in my whole life, but little did I know that the radical changes that were abut to unjustly rain down upon me were going to provide me with great blessing. How strange, for I had to be at a certain place a certain time to receive the missing link of my system. Order in Chaos, to say the least. Now my system was complete and very easy. Not hard at all, and at its core, scientific knowledge about the human body. Now I can say that I have had the opportunity to converse with "some" whom have a serious objection to knowledge. Ya, well, a certain man said his people perish because of a lack of knowledge. And so, I lost my one hundred some pounds. This is the easy sceintific method I used and the sources that explain that this scientific principle or "knowledge" is known. But don't worry, not only may the overweight or obese need this information, but some whom appear slim and trim. according to my scientific investigation, obesity may also affect the slim and trim in another way which is becoming an epidemic problem. Anyway, all you need is twenty pennies and this "knowledge" to embark upon you new journey. Cry now, laugh later. I found that with in a certain book. Love Frank Jr.. P.S. "Here I Ago Again, Wither I Win or Lose". P.S.S "I already won, I wonder can they see it or not?" ON to the dance floor: Ha, Ha, Ha and Bye.

ONE DAY

On one particular day, I sought out advice from a certain man who gave me one of the harshes talks of my life. He explained how some people just don't care. I asked surprised: "Just don't care about what!" His answer: "None of it, nor you, or what you have to say!" Boy did that hurt because I tried to help people help themselves, but I must say in some cases I find him to be right. I call it "The Doubting Betrayer Syndrome", for I believe some people will in the end windup betraying themselves. And so this is my effort to reach the people whom want to help themselves.

DISCLAIMER

This book is intended as a scientific reference volume only, not as a medical manual. Every effort has been made to ensure that the information contained in this book is accurate. However, neither the publisher nor the author is engaged in rendering professional advice or services to the individual reader. The ideas, procedures, and suggestions contained in this book are not intended as a substitute for consulting with your physician. All matters regarding your health require medical supervision. In addition with intention to incorparate as follows.

AUTHORS COMMENTS

There are so many things that I wish I could add to this document, but time will not allow it. Today is Sunday May 23rd, 2004. I used two different scales today to measure my weight. One scale said 174 pounds while and the other said 170 pounds. I will use 172 pounds as my average weight. I remember desperately trying to break the two hundred pound mark. That happened on November 19th, 2003 when I weighed in at 198 pounds. From there things went as follows: November 27th 2003 < Thanksgiving Day > I had broken my plan, December the second 2003 at 196 pounds, December the third 2003 at 195 pounds, December the fourth 2003 at 194 pounds, December the 9th 2003 at 194 pounds, December 17, 2003 at 193 pounds, December 19, 2003 at 190 pounds, January 9, 2004 at 186 pounds, January 31, 2004 at 185 pounds, February 3, 2004 at 182 pounds, February 9, 2004 at 180 pounds. I never gave up on hope! I wanted to give you a complete list of all the supplies and products that I used during my journey. That will have to wait for now. In my opinion, I could have finished this book by May 23, 2005 in a very raw state. I've been wrestling with myself about publishing this core of my research in what I consider to be an unfinished state. But then I must remember, it has been about one year for me. If someone had this data, I would have wanted it finished or not. What's so strange about the situation is that I am sitting here with a whole stack of information and fluff to add to this document. Without further ado, let me say that I use the < and > signs to insert imformation and thoughts. If you find them confusing, all you have to do is highlight the area from one sign to the next. The last thing I will say before closing this document is that the carbohydrate issue could be thought of as a ship in the water. How the body burns or accesses for use the stored carbohydrates called fat seems to be the issue. Think of the body as a ship full of fat. We want to empty the fat from the ship. Now part of the ship is above water, while another part of the ship is below water. We have to keep our ship moving because we're sailing on the course called life. Maybe we have to change our fuel from sugar to a herbal dietary supplement. Our smokestacks are the fumes that leave with the breath. But we need to get the fat out of our ship called the body. There seems to be something called a low carbohydrate diet. If we think of these type of diets as an iceberg, we know that part of the iceberg is above the water while the largest part is below. If we think of the process that we want to access as being the waterline, then we know we want the iceberg below the water. This

process is called ketosis. From what I understand, this ketosis process happends

at or below the daily intake of twenty total carbohydrates per day. This is why I

call it the waterline. First I want to remove the fat from my ship, then I want to

repair the whole in the ship.

In other words, I want to get rid of the fat first. Then after I reach my goal

weight, I want to rebuild the body starting with very light exercises. I feel that I

don't want to add muscle mass weight while trying to reduce my general mass. I

just remembered a movie I saw about a civil war ship. The designers put iron

plates on the sides of the ship at an angle so that incomming cannon balls would

bounce off. I think the movie was called Ironsides. Anyway, a smart captain of

another ship decided to aim his cannon ball shots just below the water line. And

down old Ironsides went!

CONCLUSION:

20 PENNIES A DAY SIMPLIFIED

First, you want to gather your food supply so that you will have ready foods that

you can eat < see: WHAT CAN I EAT by me >. Second, you shall put twenty pennies into a plastic zip lock bag. Third, you have to use the pennies to count your daily carbohydrate intake. Once you have used up your twenty pennies, that is the end of your maximum carbohydrate intake for the day. Fourth, you need to understand that science says that "lipolysis is the biochemical process of dissolving fat." "When you dissolve fat, it breaks down into glycerol and other fatty acids, which in turn break down into byproducts called ketones." When ketones are produced by the body, you are said to be in a state called Ketosis. You also need to know how to check yourself for ketones < see: PROOF OF KETOSIS RESEARCH by me >. Fifth, you want to weigh yourself daily and record your progression probably upon a calendar. Sixth, you want to increase your fluid intake as much as possible to help remove the ketones from your system. Also you want to increase your body temperature to promote further ketone release by the skin. Seventh, you want to help realign the spine and draw the intestines back into the intestinal cavity by doing the sitting chair exercises. These exercises will also cause you breathing volume to increase thereby aiding the release of ketones. Eighth, you want to raise your body temperature while you sleep in order to draw more ketones out of the body. Ninth, if possible you want to develop a reward system to give yourself a treat at the end of the day for your excellent effort!

JR. BUSH DAYS

"'God is Dad Bush says'"

Noting that the Declaration of Independence defines life as 'an endowment of the Creator,' President Bush, in a May 14 commencement address at Concordia University in Mequon, Wisconsin, said, 'Our worth as human beings does not depend on our health or productivity or independence or any other shifting value the world might apply. Our worth comes from bearing the image of our Maker. < villagevoice.com/nation May 19-25, 2004 >"

DOWN LOW

After I had lost 100 and a few pounds, I began to visit my friends. Long time no see. Now this one friend in particular began to make comments about how different I looked. " What have you been up to? " " What have you been doing? " The questioning became more intense. Finally I broke. I'll wanted to tell somebody. I took a deep breath and smiled. Then I did it! " I have lost 100 lbs.! " What are they going to say? Oh, that's nice. Wow, that's great. How do you feel? But no! Not this person. What I had told them was very sensitive to me. I really didn't want to go into the specifics about the amount of weight I had lost.

What did my friend say? The unthinkable. And not that I looked better fat. How about: " I can't wait to tell everybody! " Oh no! Please don't tell it! You do know how understanding they were, right? " I am going to call each and every person that I know who knows you and tell it! " I harried up and got away from this friend of mine. Then this friend began to press me about what I had done. Several conversations later, my friend became outraged and demanding. I then decided that if someone is going to tell it, it might as well be me. So here is the book. All I know is that I said the wrong thing to the right person on the down low.

WE ARE

"We are not defending, even in defense; we are on the attack!" To be obese, or to not be obese; this is now the question calling forward the responsive actions. I found out this was a "War" in April when I read "There's No Sugar-coating It: We're Losing Battle Of Bulge" in The Sun newspaper article by Kevin Cowheard.

HOW IT STARTED

My weight had ballooned near a whopping 300 pounds. It just seemed to ease up upon me. But I could see and feel it! In general, I was uneasy about the change in my structure. I was trying to eat healthy and all of that. Still my size was increasing. But my real motivation was my concern for my family members. I could see the whole weight issue as becoming a real problem. I thought to myself that this weight could be a killer. Was it real pain in my legs and back, or was it in my mind < Article: City Paper, Page 26 "MY BIG FAT AMERICAN ASS": May 19, 2004 : "Sacred Cows" The article is about a scientific experiment eating fast food everyday for 30 days to measure the results. " A few days into the experiment, Spurlock was complaining of fatigue and headaches." >? Walking from the front door of the house to the car, was I really out of breath? Maybe I was just getting old? Or maybe I was just getting older? Maybe I was just old! Should I have just given up and sat down? Did I want to run and dance again? What was I to do? If I give up to nature, what will I tell my family members if they face the same issue? Oh well, there is always the graveyard! I remember the pain of just getting out of the car. One day I said to myself: " look, you're grabbing the top of the door and falling out of the seat! " It was ridiculous.

So I began to collect my data in a scientific manor. I had been using herbs and vitamins, but none seemed to help. Why, I wondered? And why was I so tired all the time? Some of my friends began to call me lazy. This was painful. I was not lazy, but I was tired. A very strange type of tired. Too tired to do anything, and too tired not to do anything. What in the world was this all about? For my first experiment, I prepared some parsley juice and drank it. Shortly afterward, my stomach began to boil. Then a strange thing happened. I spent about two hours in the bathroom just sitting on the toilet. To my amazement, when I did leave the bathroom, my pants fell down. Fluid had been coming from everywhere. I had lost two belt notches in size using the toilet. I felt much better, but soon the weight or size came back. I tried to repeat the experiment, but no such luck. I had been studying the said affects of acid and alkaline foods upon the body. I had even become literate in the pH values of different foods and waters. But still there was no lasting effect. So I went back to the drawing board. I kept telling myself that I must try. But as time went on, my friends were becoming less understanding and more outspoken. Where was the love? Anyway, I thought I should start from a very basic point of I don't know! I don't know what food is. I don't know what food does. I don't know what food should do.

I don't know what it is that I am doing when I eat. I just don't know! So where

shall I start? What do I know? I know that I have collected something called

" fat "! So if I have fat inside my body. Stop! What is fat? I don't know!

FAT EXPERIMENT

I went to the refrigerator and grabbed a pot with meat in it. Look, that hard white

stuff on top. I broke off two large pieces. I went and got two jars. I put a piece

of the white stuff in each jar. I then put water in each jar and placed them in the

refrigerator. I then took some of the fat and put it in a pan on the stove. I heated

the pan and watched the "fat" liquefy. I then put that melted fat in a third jar in

the refrigerator. I came back later to find the clear liquid " fat " had returned to a

hard and white state. What conclusions could I draw? My hypothesis were these:

1) since the human body was closer to the temperature of the heated pan, the " fat

" in my body might be in a liquid state; 2) due to some unknown reason, " fat " in

general would collect together. Now, if this " fat " would collect, it might also

collect on the veins and arteries walls blocking nutrients from getting to and into

my organs. What could I do about this fat? But wait a minute, I have not been

eating " fat "!

SWEETIE

I had read the book " The Sugar Blues " by William Dufty a few years back. I had long ago cut back on sugar < so I thought >. But I did notice, if I slipped an began to eat sweets, boy would I eat sweets. Six doughnuts, no problem; until I finished eating them. I could watch myself gobble down four or six at a time. To be truthful, really six or eight doughnuts. But afterwards I always felt guilty and worse. Now I am being accused of being greedy. How in the hell can I be greedy with my own doughnuts? These people? Why are there comments so negative? I feel myself drowning, and what do they do? They throw me bricks. I must help myself! I can help myself! I, me, us, and we are the only ones that are going to help me. I am all alone. Where is the love? Maybe it is not " fat " but sugar? What do I know about sugar? Nothing. So, I brought a piece of sugar cane. Wait just a minute. I licked the sugar cane and was surprised. The sugar cane was weak compared to white granule sugar in taste. I then chopped up the sugar cane and put the pieces into the blender with water. I drank the sugar cane water mixture. It was weak. I wondered how many sugar canes does it take to make one teaspoon of sugar? I still don't know! But I had cut down my sugar consumption, so I thought. I also did an experiment with sugar. I put some crystal sugar in a pan.

I added water to the sugar and watched it turn into a liquid. I then put the pan into the oven. After the water had evaporated, the crystal sugar was left in the pan. What was my hypothesis? Maybe it is liquefied sugar in my system, and it is clumping together like the fat. So what? I want to get what ever it is out of my system. Suppose if it is fat and sugar? How can I get it out of my " pipes " if it has grouped together in a liquid state? I need a cutter. What cuts through grease? Lemons? Why do they call it lemonade? What is the "aid " part? Stop! Don't they put sugar in lemonade? Yes. So I began to think of lemons and water. I then conducted the fat in the jar experiment with lemon juice. I did not see a change in the fat. Besides, I was aware of the drink eight glasses of water a day theory. Now I had to be true to myself. I was not drinking eight glasses of water now. Would I drink the eight glasses of water with lemon juice? No! Like a child I said to myself: "I don't like it ". I could see this whole process as being a big misery. I am all ready miserable. So what? I still have to try. < HONEY: Egyptians were the first people known to keep bees. Honey was collected to sweeten cakes, beer, and wine. < Back Packs Books: 1001 Facts About Ancient Egypt: Page 48: Scott Steedman >>

ALCOHOL

What could I use to cut the bonding process of fat and sugar? Maybe I need a

solvent? Well, that is a nice term, but what could I use? I had no idea. I thought

and thought about it. I did not have a clue. Then one day I saw a bottle of rubbing

alcohol sitting on a table. Alcohol < Page 2F: The Sun April 14, 2004 : " Health

News That's Worthy Of A Toast" : " Alcohol In Moderation Can Help, Study

Says " > ! My mind said to me that alcohol is a solvent. What? Yes, it also

cleans like when doctors use it in surgery I thought. Being familiar with martial

arts, I thought of the drunken style of Kung Fu. But in the movies about Shaolin

Temple, when someone would ask about " the drunken style ", the instructors

would say: " there is no drunken Kung Fu!" But there he was, an old master

drinking wines and eating whole roasted chickens. Now this was very strange.

You say there is no drunkard Kung Fu, but there is an old master drinking wine

and eating meat? I have watched martial arts movies. I had seen the drunkard

master in those movies! I was also aware of Buddah Damo, He was the black

Indian monk who is said to have taught the monks at Shaolin Temple a certain set

of moves. It was said that the monks had become so physically weak from

practicing spiritual Zen meditation that they could barely move. Damo is said to

have meditated for ten years in front of a rock before teaching the monks the

moves or forms.

Why, I asked myself? To become as the monks were! So I assumed that he had meditated in a fixed posture until his body became weak like the monks bodies. Then he devised the postures and exercises to recover his physical strength. Wait, is this not in the Bible also? Did Adam and Eve " eat " something that they knew not what it was? Did that food change them? Strange, Damo is from India, which is in Asia. The Book of the Revelation speaks to seven churches in Asia! Wine? Is not wine used in The Bible? So I began to experiment with wines and alcohol. I did my fat in the jar test. Yes, the fat broke apart. The fat in the jar with alcohol looked different than with lemon juice.

STRANGERS

I happen to meet two sets of people whom were very helpful. Christi and Skip heard my cries for help and spoke firmly to me about moving forward. And I thank you! Keith and Jeremy noticed that I was doing strange movements and inquired if I was trying to lose weight or exercise. I was doing both! "One Thousand Strokes of the Chinabar" < part of and upcoming work in progress titled: "Kundalinion Sexual Tantra : One Thousand Strokes Of The Chinabar" > I called my exercises. Taking a clue from Damo, I devised specific exercises to help my back and stomach. I started the exercise sitting in a chair on my front porch. Basically, I would rock back and forth one thousand times. I would contract my stomach and stretch my back. I was given this tip by Master Garcia Davis of the Champions martial arts organization. The group was headed by Grand Master L. R. Butcher Sr.. In developing these special exercises, Grand Master Butcher had specifically told me to " not burn out the body "! He explained that I wanted to warm up the body, but not exhaust myself while in a weaken state. He even explained that if I overwork or shocked the body, it would rebel against the activity with pain. I found out the hard way that he was right. So, I choreographed the exercises to be easy and simple.

Once I worked my way up to ten thousand movements in the chair, I changed to standing exercises of the same nature. But I did feel that I had made one wrong assumption. You see that done lap? You know, when your stomach done lapped over your belt. You know, what they call " fat ". Well, I don't think that is " fat "! I think your intestines have swollen and fallen out of the midsection cavity. That's not fat, that's your intestines I said to myself. Suck it in as you were told. So I was in the beginning stages of this when Keith and Jeremy inquired about my behavior. Jeremy and Keith had knowledge of Dr. Atkins. Jeremy explained to me how his parents had lost a few pounds using Dr. Atkins concept. Jeremy had never used the Atkins concept. Keith, on the other hand, had used the concept to lose five pounds or so. Yah right! My problem was about one hundred pounds!

Not ten, not twenty, not fifty; but one hundred pounds! I reviewed Dr. Atkins information anyway. I remember a flash of sudden insight. What, carbohydrates turned into sugar in the body? But what do you call the sugars of the body? I remember a test I had taken years ago. " Glucose!" Glucose, isn't that related to insulin? Doesn't glucose turn to alcohol in the brain? I am still not sure, but I think I had heard this information. Then in a strange turn of events, Keith books a trip for the summer. So? So, he needs to drop a few pounds now. But summer is so far off. Yes, but as part of the celebration in looking forward to the trip, Keith wants to lose a few pounds now. How? He is going to do his Atkins thing.

So Keith announces that he is about to drop a few pounds. Then he asks if anyone wants to join him. He explains that he would enjoy the company. Yes, that is me! I asked him why he would want company on a weight loss program? He explained how two or more people can relate to each other and be supportive. I didn't really understand how, but I was for trying. What did Keith do? He showed me his food. Keith had already started before he made it known what he was doing. Maybe it was to prepare those around him for the change in his behavior. "See!" " See my lunch", Keith said? Yah, right! So the next day I was eating my special food. I was eating some fried chicken when Keith walked into the room. He asked if I was eating lunch? I said yes! I was very happy to say "yes "! Then he swiftly walked away. He returned with a huge soda and threw it at me. Now I am puzzled. A soda on a low carbohydrate diet? Before I could speak, Keith asked me what I was eating again? I replied " fried chicken "! Here the egos come! He then said in a demanding voice: " drink the soda ". He spoke to me as if I were Judas Iscariot himself. I must admit I had a few choice thoughts about Keith, but I caught myself. Humbly I asked, " what is wrong with my lunch?" Keith asked again, " what is that?" Again I said " fried chicken". Then I went on to explain how there were no carbohydrates in chicken. You see, I am an expert now! Yah right! Keith began yelling about how dumb and stupid I was. Boy, how Keith my former friend, among other things, was cutting into me.

I was becoming emotional now! I am thinking of words that start with certain letters. Now who does Keith go and get? Jeremy! Here they come. Jeremy looked at my lunch, and the two fell out in laughter. I want to know. All I want to know is: what in the Sam Hill is so damned funny? So I asked about the nature of their laughter? " It's the skin on your chicken!" The skin? "Yes, your zero carbohydrate chicken is soaked in batter." "And what is batter", Keith asked? I am Mr. Dummy. That is bread, or flour; and they are both carbohydrates. So I drank the soda. Later Keith explained how he had gone through the same thing. He wanted me to remember the event and added that I would do better with a rotisserie chicken tomorrow. So the next day I went to the supermarket and brought a whole chicken for lunch. Then Keith explained that the same thing had happened to him with his first buddy. Thank you Keith, Jeremy, Christi and Skip! Well, Keith lost his few pounds and said we should celebrate. Yah right! I asked: "What are we going to have, some bottled water from France"? " No ", he said: "We are going to have a beer". I fell out laughing, "A beer?" "Yes", Keith replied. "A new low carbohydrate beer of about two carbs!" "How many?" "Two or three each beer", Keith said. I really started laughing. Then I began to dance! Oh Happy day. It was around May 2003. I had not lost much weight. As a matter of fact, I weighed 283 pounds on the industrial scale a month or so earlier. To be accurate, about one month and a belt notch smaller. But I had a plan. Big fat, fat ass lazy Frank.

THE PLAN

How should I go about this weight loss issue? First of all, I don't want to work hard. I have my exercises that I can even do in the car. I assumed that if the carbohydrates turned to sugar in my system, then I have about one hundred pounds of carbohydrates with me at all times. The exercises < as approved by Master Edward Butcher Sr. and Master Edward Butcher Jr. of the Champions >

will help to stimulate fluid movement < as agreed upon by Master Sonny Butcher, Jr. in reference to the use of beer > in my system, lightly work the muscle groups, and allow me time to work on my breathing. Breathing will become a special part of my plan. When will I reward myself? After I exercise. I will drink the low carbohydrate beer as part of my reward system. Now, I will begin to associate the reward with the work! How many beers can I have per day? I will deal with that in a little while. Alright, I have a light exercise to do, and the great reward of a low carbohydrate beer. What else will I do? I will go outside to do my chair exercises so that I get fresh air and sunlight. I had read that sunlight turns to vitamin " D " in the body. This also may help to counter act what is called seasonal disorder. Which brings me to the concept of sleep < Article: U. S. News & World Report, May 17, 2004 Page 58 "The Secrets Of Sleep".

"Sleep is clearly important – after all, people and animals slumber away a third of their lives – but no one knows why." "What's more, experiments that deprived animals of REM sleep by disrupting them during this sleep stage found that they didn't learn as well as animals that got plenty of dreaming." "'It's frankly the only biological role for sleep that makes much sense for me,' says Stickgold." "Researchers can point to a whole list of diseases connected to sleep deprivation." "Inadequate sleep comes with a high cost. Perhaps the most graphic example of the link between sleep and illness is bipolar disorder, or manic-depression. ' I've always believed the mania caused the lack of sleep, and the lack of sleep

worsened the mania,' says Alexis." "' And mania is preceded by an episode of

insomnia' says Ruth Benca, a professor of psychiatry at the University of

Wisconsin." > < Note to myself: put your headphones on please, because " the

cicadas " just have to keep making noise, any noise, all noise while they can

clearly see that you are trying to THINK! Oh no, noise etc. I just could not figure

out what was wrong. "An authors environment is so very important, as with

interrupting their thinking process by making that noise. I am THINKING!">

< Article: U. S. News & World Report, May 17, 2004 Page 71 " A Nation's

Wake-up Call ". " Everyone should be a student of sleep, most especially one's

own."

" Babies emerge from the darkness of the womb sleeping some 16 hours a day."

>. Now if my body is burning fat, it could be considered as having done a

chemical work out. If the reduction in weight comes from physical or chemical

work, work is being done. So whether the work is done by chemical or physical

means, the body needs recovery time. So I figured I would need a lot of rest. In

my first book, Baptist Gnostic Christian Eubonic Kundalinion Spiritual Ki Do

Hermeneutic Metaphysics ISBN # 0-595-20678-6, I discussed something I called

"Kundalion Hibernation ". I have decided that I would try to keep the body warm

at all times while I sleep. My concept is that perspiration would aid in the weight loss. I then decided to wear a thick hooded sweat suit to bed at night. Yes I put the hood on my head. I had read that heat and magnetic current was lost through the uncovered head. I had purchased four different color sweat suits, but little did I know how much I would use them! Once on the way with my system, I found I might change the sweat suit twice per night. I was often awakened from my sleep by the damp or wet clothes. Yes my system was putting out water, but so what? Dehydration became an issue. I decided to also do breathing exercises while I was in bed. No, I am not watching the television. I am worried about my breath intake and output. Remember the beer intake. I see the beer as being high in water. I also decided to increase my water intake. I drank as much water as I could. I put a glass in the bathroom. I drank water every time I went to the bathroom. Speaking of being in the bathroom, I tried to use the bathroom as a tool. I would stay in the bathroom for about two hours. First I would turn on a compact disk. Next I would get into the tub and turn the shower on. I used the shower to fill the tub while I was standing up. So in a way, I was soaking my feet. I might stop the shower and lather up with soap. Then I would wash it off. My concept was to open my pores and degrease my skin. I also hoped to increase the elasticity of my skin. The heat from the water also may help to liquefy the fat and sugar. So while the shower was running and the compact disc was playing; I would dance and exercise in the tub. I decided that I should incorporate dancing into my exercise system. I began to return to the disco. All I can say is: "dance and sit down, dance and sit down, and dance and sit down". But my concept is the easy does it! Sure you can work yourself to death, but easy does it. Just like the weight eased up on me, I want to ease up upon the weight! Easy does it, easy does it with beer and meat. While on the subject of the bathroom, I had begun to watch my urine. This became important. Oh, while in the tub, after the shower part; I would work my fingers and toes. Yes, clean and cut your toenails. Wiggle this little pig, which are your toes. I would press the toenail to increase the blood movement under the nail! My concept was that every little bit helps! I had learned about nail pressing from Tai Chi practice. What about emergency sugar attacks? Well, I felt I must keep low carbohydrate snacks are around at all times.

One night, to my surprise, I had a sugar attack. No big deal. I had a bag of low carbohydrate jellybeans. I sat on the bed and ate the whole bag. So what? The next day I sat upon the toilet a long time. All I can say is that I have not done that again. But always be ready for any emergency sugar attack. Go now and by emergency low sugar snacks. Go now I thought to myself. So I did it. I then came to believe that snacks and treats are not like food! So what should I do? How about buying large bags of cheese and multiple rotisserie chickens. If I could have, I would have kept eight chickens in the freezer. Eat, eat, eat and never ever be hungry. Keep it simple! Yes, but suppose it is the midday? Go to the salad bar and you know what to do! Go low on those carbs! I began to remind myself as to which foods were lowest in carbohydrates! Strange how soon afterwards some of my friends began to be diagnosed with " sugar diabetes ". When I was a child, it was called " sugar "! I had read that the ancient doctors called shamen would taste the patients urine. If the urine was sweet, they would say " sugar "! Can you imagine that? What about the meat I was consuming? I figured that I wanted ground meat so that it would be easy upon my intestines for digestion and the release of energy. So, I would prepare my food in the microwave oven in a dish with water. Maybe water was being drawn into my intestines to hydrate the meal. Well. I started cooking with water. Now it was not the best tasting, but with some help from cheese and special herbs, the meals were not that bad!

I did begin to notice that some cans of foods listed the sugar and carbohydrate counts. Many times they were equal, and most times they were close to each other. When the can said "X" number of carbohydrate grams, I began to think of "X" grams of sugar. Grams, what is that? Meter, liter, and gram, how do I convert them into pounds? I looked up gram in the dictionary and did the calculations. So what if I ate "X" number of grams of carbohydrates? I assumed that I had an increase in my body weight by the converted calculated amount above my normal which equaled one hundred pounds. I may be beginning to understand this weight issue! So carbohydrates equal sugar, which equals weight to be stored in the body. Want about my intestines? I had read information about the intestines being clogged. I decided to use an old time remedy to clean my intestines out.

On one occasion I drank a whole jug of prune juice, and on another I ate a whole loaf of raisin bread. The result of doing both was sitting upon the toilet a long time. And while I am on the subject of parts falling off and out, what is that falling off my arm? You know how that meat hangs from under the arm, what is that: fat? Half way through my experiment, I noticed that when I made a muscle, the "fat" moved from under my arm to the side. Wait a minute. That's not fat, that is my muscle! I believe that my whole muscle had fallen off the upper bone of my arm! This is a whole new definition of falling apart. I must change my life style and knowledge of the workings of the human body verses just doing a diet!

MIRROR MIRROR LIE

When will I start my new " diet " concept? I do not know! Then it happened. Have you ever flushed the toilet only to find waste still in the bowl? I did, but I had to wait for the tank to refill with water. I began to walk away. I had flushed the toilet, oh I need to flush it again! So I went back to flush the toilet again. Then

I walked away from the second flush. Everyday I had looked in the mirror. Yes, I looked just fine. Today, yesterday, and the day before that I looked just fine. In the mirror I looked fine. So as I began to walk away from the toilet for the second time, I passed by my trusty mirror. No I did not stop to look, but I did check myself. I turned my head slightly to say yes and kept walking. I took about two steps and thought: "who was that? "? Back up! Wow, who is that? I turned forward and looked at my face. It was me in the mirror. Then I turned to the side and moved away to get a full view. Oh no, why didn't anyone tell me?

HOUSE OF DRACULA

I began to run around my house. I was looking for a full length mirror. Who moved all the mirrors? Who lives here? Is it the living dead? Whose house doesn't have mirrors? Oh that is easy. It is Dracula the undead who has no mirrors. I need to see myself! There are no full length mirrors in this house. I have one in the basement. I had walked past the mirror in the bathroom without a shirt on and seen something I had never seen before. Who is that? I ran to my basement and dug out a mirror panel! I pulled out the mirror and got bone naked. What is that? Who is that? And from the rear, we won't even discuss that! Oh no, today must be the day! That is not me! I know me! That is not, is not me!

Just look at that, me! No more time. Today is the date. What about what I don't know? Damn that, this is life! This is about life! This is about my life. One day I will be dead, but today I live. And as I live, and as I see, for my eyes are open. I do see. Yes my friends will be with me. Major wrong! Today is the day! There is no tomorrow, today is day one. I gave myself a harsh pep talk. It wasn't so nice. This was it. I am at the fork in the road. Real funny, a fork! You know what I mean. It is the point of no return! It is the last day. Judgment Day! Do or die! But I do have hope! Yes, I have done research. Am I ready?

All I have is what I have. I believe in God, and so onto the battlefield of life I go. I may have to leave the friends I know behind. So goodbye! But I will not go out as a sissy!

KETOSIS CONCEPT

While reviewing Dr. Atkins research, I noticed different levels on the carbohydrate intakes. Sometimes twenty grams, sometimes forty grams, and sometimes higher. Twenty grams of carbohydrate verses zero I thought. Yes, maybe I could kick in the ketosis process with zero carbohydrates. In my opinion, I was one hundred pounds way over weight. That is several ounces and several grams of carbohydrates. I carry these carbohydrates around with me and

all times. Two hundred and eighty three pounds " plus ". Yes, it is time to do or
die so to speak.

DAY ONE

On day one I began to start upon my new adventure! All my ideas and concepts
being activated as one. Did I receive help from those friends close to me? No! I
was acting weird. Oh, weird big, big fat, fat ass Frank. Yah well, who is Frank?
Not that person I saw in the mirror. "Oh heck no", I cried inside myself. No time
for crying. Today is day one. Stick to the plan no matter what. Yes I did that.
How was the year? To say " terrible " would be mild! As strange as it may
seem, I saw one sickness leave me, while I saw another sickness come towards
me. The truth is sometimes sad, very sad. I saw some so called friends act very
ugly. Really ugly! But I did not let them throw me off my plan. And yes it was
hard. But I kept on with the plan. From mid May 2003 at two hundred eighty
three plus pounds, yes plus pounds; to one hundred eighty pounds on February
9,2004. Oh ya, and when I put on those size thirty-three waist jeans; I laughed?
All I wondered about at that moment was what was I laughing about?

FRANK M. CONAWAY, JR.

LET ME SEE

This is how it all seemed to come together. I had been studying several areas of science dealing with the human body. I had been aware of mine increase in weight for some years. Call it the mythological high school weight syndrom if you will. You know when someone wishes they could be the size they were in high school. Well, my waist size was about 34 inches. My weight was 165 pounds at best. This was my competition weight in Karate tournaments. So for years I had dreamed of these figures. Well, a twenty year dream liken to an odyssey! I had tried many concepts over the years, only to fail. But I always kept hope within my heart! Fail I might, but I always kept hope. I would say that one day I would get my weight issue under control. Then I might add five or ten pounds. Two pounds here, one pound there; and one day you get a surprise in the mirror. I got my surprise shortly after Keith had finished his weight loss. It all happened at once. It seems as if Keith had received his reward an finished, while I was about to begin. But what Keith and I were doing just was not working for me. I didn't know why! It just wasn't happening. Maybe I was looking for a physical change and thereby was able to " see " myself in the mirror. Once I did, I formulated a plan using " all " the knowledge I had at the time. I decided to zero out my carbohydrate intake for at least three miserable days. I've decided to increase my water intake. But how would I know how much water I was drinking per day. Well, the first three days it really didn't matter. But then I came up with this great idea. I can track my water consumption by using the beer bottles. It became very basic to me. It was "a" or "b". "A" was water or unsweetened tea may be with lemon juice in a beer bottle. "B" was of course a nice cold beer. I had studied about the affects colored glass has upon liquids, and I thought the bottles shaped would give the water a spin rate. So I could wash the empty bottles, soak off the labels, filled them with water or mild tea, cool them in the refrigerator in the six pack case, and returned the empty bottles to the counters six-pack cases for cleaning and refill. What a great system, and I could tell the water or tea bottles from the beer bottles because of the missing labels. Oh no, no one else could. Shortly after I started with my " whole " concept, I had some friends visit me. I guess they were wondering where I had been. Well, you can collect a lot of beer bottles in four to six weeks. On one hand time just slips by. Yes the one hand it goes fast, but on the other the daily temptation makes it seem twice as long. Anyway, here come my friends to visit me. They sure would like something to drink. Hey, would you like a beer? And there it was! Ninety-nine bottles of beer on the wall! I am looking at my friends and they are looking at my beer bottles.

Let's see, empty beer bottles soaking in water to remove the labels, empty clean

beer bottles on the counter ready to be refilled with liquid, clean and dry beer

bottle tops in a bowl, empty beer bottles in the six pack case to be counted for my

liquid consumption total waiting to be cleaned, and beer bottles in the refrigerator

with water, tea, or beer in them. Now I am not going to give my friends in a

bottle of water in a beer bottle! So, I ask: "Would you like a glass of water?"

One friend asks for a soda. Oh, I have no soda! Now, would you like water or

beer? Well, one friend says beer. Here it comes. I opened the refrigerator and

their may be twenty-four beer bottles in there. In reality, there may have been

more. So how many beer bottles are we talking about? Let's count them. How

about six sixpacks < two at water, two at tea, two at beer > or thirty-six bottles in

the refrigerator, twelve bottles on the counter, six bottles in the sink, eight bottles

on the dish dryer, and two sealed twelve packs < that's twenty-four bottles > on

the floor waiting to be chilled! How many beer bottles is this? What's the

problem? I had taken my concepts down to what I called a basic level. So you've

opened the refrigerator and what do you see? Thirty-six brown bottles in six-pack

cases, three whole rotisserie chickens, four jars of pickles, maybe one jar of

pickle juice, four packages of cheese, three packages of bacon, three boxes of

eggs, two bottles of hot sauce, and a bowl of ten cooked hamburgers. How

simple. Really, I had three different sections of " beer bottles" in the refrigerator.

One section was plain water, while another was tea with lemond juice. I also thought of the lemond juice as being a degreeser. The third section was for beer. Oh, over on the counter near the bowl of beer bottle caps, I kept two bottles of lemon juice concentrate and three bottles of spices in water. What's so wrong about this picture? There I am. I am wearing a bright orange hooded sweat suit standing in front of this scene. Well, to ease the tension I asked if anyone would like some chicken with their beer? Strange looks is what I got! One friend asked:" And what have you been doing Frank? " " Oh, I have been resting! " " It's about seven p.m. and I have been resting. " "So where have you been? " Then someone had to use the bathroom.

DOOR NUMBER THREE

The front door that my friends came in through was door number one. The refrigerator door was door number two. And now there it was, door number three. Let me just tell you how it happend. When the bathroom door was opened, out came the strong smell of bleach. Cut on the light switch and the radio automatically comes on. Ah, it was what you call a boom box. The boom box had detachable cube like speakers. Now the boom box is angled across the handbowl so the music gives me a nice acoustical affect while I am in the tub.

There are about fifteen CDs on top of the boom box. You see, if I play one whole CD, that would equal about one hour and a half of time spent in the bathroom. I also had about five cassette tapes to choose from. Let me put it to you like this. You opened the bathroom door to the strong smell of plastic shower curtains soaking in bleach and you see: a shower with the curtains soaking in the tub, one large boom box upon the handbowl, fifteen CDs, five cassette tapes, two or three types of toothpaste, two very large bottles of mouthwash, two electric toothbrushes on chargers, two hand held toothbrushes, three different cans of air fresheners, four or five packages of incense, one incense holder, a book of matches, a lighter, one oil incense burner sitting upon a ceramic dish with its special candles beside it, two or three different bottles of incense oil, seven or so packages of shaving razors, three different types of scissors, three types of nail clippers, one cordless electric shaver on charge, five different types of skin lotion, a bottle of lemon juice for my bath water, two bottles of that bath bubbles, two large jugs of beach, one bottle of pine oil cleaner, a couple packages of toilet deodorizer, two types of toilet bowl cleaner, four or five boxes of hand soap, one large body sponge, two nail files, several metal tools for cleaning under the nails, one dead skin foot rock, three or four packages of facial clay, one set of electric hair clippers, one bottle of glass cleaner, one bottle of tile scum remover, eight rolls of toilet tissue, one electric air cleaner, a few magazines, one cordless electric hair clipper, one skin brush and back washer, a inflatable bathtub neck

pillow, a inflatable bathtub back cushion, one shower cap, one pair of dark

sunglasses, one bottle of tooth polish, two pair of tweezers, one straight razor,

two electric hair dryers, two different types of hair brushes, one drinking glass,

two or three cans of shaving cream, one electric foot soaker massager, two or

three cans of foot spray, one spray bottle with oil in it, about five washcloths,

three large towels, one toilet brush, one shower curtain brush, one sink cleaning

brush, one sponge for cleaning the mirror, one set of flip flops, one robe, one

black light, one hand held mirror, one wash mitten, one can of oven cleaner, one

mug by the tub to pour water upon myself, one bottle of peroxide, two bottles of

rubbing alcohol, one can of hair sheen spray, two different colored sponge balls,

one big red rubber hot water bottle, three boxes of epsom salt, one plastic bag of

tooth flossers, one cordless electric tooth flosser on its charger with extra heads,

one water jet system, one box of plastic bags, one trashcan, one box of trashcan

trash bags, one bag of cotton balls in a plastic bag, one bottle of nail polish

remover, about twenty pennies in a clear glass, one wire egg beater, one bottle of

clear nail polish, one small reading lamp, two cans of cleaning powder, one

plunger, one bucket and mop, a few bottles of cologne, one flashlight, one fly

swatter, two large industrial rubber gloves, one backbrace that looked like a

girdle, one set of garggles, one box of tissues, one metal hair pick, one plastic comb, two plastic hair picks, two ink pens and a small pad, one pad of sticky

labels, a few highlighters, about six different clear plastic bags of dried flowers

for the tub with a strainer bag, one floating book stand, one net pool bag, a candle

holder with several scented candles, one digital thermometer, one sauna suit, one

pair of pool shoes, one pair of swimming trunks, one nail buffer, two plastic balls

for hand exercises, one anti slip tub mat, one scalp massager, one small fan, one

empty glass pickle jar with top, one box of baking soda, one box of cue tips, a

few plastic hooks on suction cups, one screwdriver, one clear box of colored

paper clips, one shower cap, one nose cleaning jar, one tongue scraper, one

lighted two sided facial mirror, one pillowcase with the zipper, one soap on a

rope, one box of suppositories, one bottle of witch hazel, and one plastic tugboat

with captains whistle! Maybe it was the blow up neck pillow that did it?

I just don't think that they understood! I just don't think my friends were thinking

of function and form! And there it was! Now put me in a very thick hooded bright

orange sweat suit together with the kitchen and bathroom sceen. But what is so

strange about it I asked you? I also remember the comments made at the liquor

store when I started buying the low carbohydrate beer. At first most stores didn't

have it. I would get strange looks and remarks. Most people said that the beer

was like water! How could I explain the sugar factor. As far as the bathroom is

concerned, I think of the whole issue as being hygienic! Well, at least no one said

I was stinky Frank! As I see it, the only strange thing was the black light in the bathroom < maybe / maybe not > . You would be surprised at what you see in the bathroom under the black light.

NO HIGH

Is it not upon the label, "high fructose corn syrup sugar"! You don't want that, although it tastes "good" to the mouth but not unto the loins, it is as yeast! Hear this, and reject or choose your way, by knowledge of and by there of!

DOING WRONG

Sometimes you just do what you should not. Be truthful with yourself. It might be painful, but it is what it is. For example, check your height to weight ratio. For it is one thing to be overweight, and another to be obese. You might need this knowledge in particular. When losing weight and acting strange, you might be confronted with the perception that you are losing too much weight. I know because it happened to me. The more I tried to explain what my goals were, the more it was explained to me how I was becoming too small. I just could not stop the helpful criticism. But then, painful as it was, I had to confess that according to the doctor's charts on height to weight ratios, I was obese. "But you will."

Please, the medical charts say that I am obese. Well, how much more? The

medical charts say that I am obese. Really, which one it is worse: to look obese,

to be obese, to look and be obese, or not to look obese but to be obese? To be or

not to be, is that the question. "Be honest with yourself." "**Obesity:** WHAT IS

IT? Obesity is conventionally defined as an excess of stored fat resulting in a

body weight that is 20 percent or greater than what is accepted as ideal for a

person's height and body type. Though not itself a disease, obesity is a serious

health risk. Mortality rates and the incidence of high blood pressure, coronary

heart disease, and diabetes mellitus are substantially higher in obese adults,

especially in those whose excessive fat is stored in the abdomen rather than in the

hips. Excess weight increases the risk of gallbladder disease and may cause or

aggravate arthritis by placing greater stress on the back, hips, and knees. Certain

types of cancer in may also be more common in overweight people. In addition,

obesity is often accompanied by poor self-image, psychological distress, and

diminished quality of life. Losing weight and keeping it off, however, is

extraordinarily difficult.

WHAT CAUSES IT? Obesity results from an imbalance between caloric intake

and energy expenditure, usually due to habitually excessive food intake and/or

limited physical activity. Some people may gain weight because they have lower basal metabolic rates: they burn fewer calories to maintain body functions, such as breathing, heart contractions, and digestion. Hereditary, environmental, and psychological factors all play a role in obesity.

PREVENTION Establish healthy eating habits; maintain a nutritious, low-fat, high-carbohydrate diet. < Source: Johns Hopkins Symptoms And Remedies: Medical Editor Simeon Margolis, M. D.,Ph. D. >" < **Obesity:** A condition in which there is an accumulation of access body fat.

AGE More common with increasing age

GENDER More Common in females GENETICS Sometimes runs in families LIFESTYLE Overeating and a sedentary lifestyle are risk factors

A person is considered obese if he or she weighs at least 20 percent more than the maximum healthy weight for his or her height (see: ARE YOU A HEALTHY WEIGHT?, P.53). About 3 in 10 people in the US are obese, and the condition is becoming increasingly common. Obesity can cause many health problems due to the strain it puts on organs and joints. For example, back pain, painful hips and knees, and shortness of breath are common problems. Obesity increases the risk of some widespread and potentially fatal disorders, such as coronary artery disease (P.405), stroke (p.532), and high blood pressure (see: HYPERTENSION, p.403). Obesity may also lead to psychological problems, including depression (p.554). WHAT ARE THE CAUSES? Obesity occurs when food taken into the body provides more energy than is used. The main causes are overeating and a sedentary lifestyle. Obesity may run in families as a result of learned' eating habits as well as inherited factors. In rare cases, obesity may be a symptom of a hormonal disorder, such as hypothyroidism (p.680). Some drugs, especially corticosteroids (p.930), can also lead to obesity. Occasionally, obesity may be a result of a psychological problem.

ARE THERE COMPLICATIONS? Obesity increases the risk of various chronic health problems. For example, obese people are more likely to have high blood cholesterol levels (see: HYPERCHOLESTEROLEMIA, p.69 1).

High cholesterol in turn increases the risk of atherosclerosis (p.402), in which fatty deposits build up on the inner linings of the arteries. Atherosclerosis may contribute to high blood pressure, coronary artery disease, and strokes. Arterial thrombosis and embolism (p.431), which is blockage of a blood vessel by a blood clot, occurs more often in obese people. Obese adults are at greater risk of gallstones (p.651) and are more likely to develop diabetes mellitus (p.687). Certain cancers, such as prostate cancer (p.726), breast cancer (p.759), and cancer of the uterus (p.748), are also more common in obese people. Excess weight can put strain on joints. Osteoarthritis (p.374) is common in obese people, especially in the hips and knees. Sleep apnea (p.477), a respiratory disorder, is also associated with obesity.

WHAT MIGHT BE DONE? Your doctor will probably measure your weight and height and discuss your diet with you (see: A HEALTHY DIET, p.48). He or she will probably also ask you how much exercise you do (see: EXERCISE AND HEALTH, pp.55-61). Tests may be performed to measure blood sugar levels (to look for diabetes) and cholesterol levels (see: BLOOD CHOLESTEROL TESTS, p.231). Rarely, you may have blood tests to check for a hormonal disorder. Obesity is most commonly treated by a weight-reduction diet and increased exercise.

Calorie intake per day is usually reduced to 500-1,000 calories less than the average requirement for a person of your age, sex, and height (see: CONTROLLING YOUR WEIGHT, p.53,). This type of eating plan is designed to produce slow, sustainable weight loss. The diet may be formulated by your doctor or a dietitian, although you may also choose to join a self-help group. Moderate and regular exercise is essential in losing weight. Appetite suppressant drugs are available but many are not recommended because of side effects. However, newer drugs with fewer side effects are under development. Sibutramine controls the appetite by affecting neurotransmitters in the brain. Drugs that reduce fat absorption from the digestive tract, such as orlistat, may also help. Rarely, surgery is used to treat obesity. For example, the stomach may be stapled to reduce its size so that you feel full after small meals. Changes in diet and lifestyle need to be maintained throughout life. Support from your family, doctor, and a selfhelp group should help you follow your weight-loss plan successfully. < Source: American College Of Physicians Complete Home Medical Guide: Editor-In-Chief David R. Goldman, MD FACP page 631 >> "

" < YOUR BODY AND DISEASE Mental problems due to physical illness One or more psychological conditions resulting from a physical illness

LIFESTYLE Unsettled domestic or financial circumstances are risk factors

AGE GENDER GENETICS Not significant factors Changes in mental state are a common response to a physical illness.

A serious physical illness may cause anxiety (see: ANXIETY DISORDERS, p.551), depression (P.554), anger, or denial of the problem. Usually, reactions are transient and resolve when the person adjusts to the change in his or her physical condition. However, illnesses that may be fatal or chronic disorders that involve lengthy treatment or continued disability may cause persistent mood problems. People who have had previous psychiatric disorders are more at risk, as are people who are subject to additional stresses, such as an unstable home life or financial problems or who generally find it hard to deal with adversity. Mood problems are sometimes a recognized svmptom of a physical illness. For example, anxiety is a svmptom of the hormonal disorder hvperthvroidism (p.679), and depression is associated with multiple sclerosis (p.541) and also Parkinson's disease (see PARKINSON'S DISEASE AND PARKINSONISM, p.539).

WHAT ARE THE SYNIPTOMS? The psychological symptoms that may result from a physical illness include: Feelings of anxiety, ranging from mild apprehension to fear and panic. Depressive symptoms, such as loss of interest and hopelessness. Irritability and anger. In extreme cases, there may be social withdrawal and drug or alcohol abuse.

WHAT MIGHT BE DONE? If the doctor thinks you are at risk of developing a psychological problem as a result of illness, you will be offered support and counseling (p.971) to help you adjust. If there are signs that you are a voiding coming to terms with an illness, the doctor will encourage you to ask questions and talk about possible anxieties. Home and work problems may be discussed, and the doctor will want to know if you have a history of depression or anxiety disorders. A person who has developed psychological problems as a result of illness may not be aware of it, and a family member or friend may be the first to contact the doctor. An antidepressant medication (p.916) or, less commonly, an antianxiety medication (p.916) may be prescribed for a short time. The person may be referred to a psychiatrist, who will encourage a problem-solving approach to the physical illness that concentrates on developing solutions rather than

focusing on difficulties. The prognosis for a mental problem resulting from

physical illness depends on a person's ability to cope with the demands of his or

her illness and its severity. Given continued support, most people are able to

recognize and deal with mood problems and find that they gradually diminish as a

result. < Source: American College Of Physicians Complete Home Medical

Guide: Editor-In-Chief David R. Goldmann, MD FACP Page 558 >"

THROWING IT OUT

Don't play around with your health. I remember the day I started on my new
plan. I had just purchased a six pack of clear soda. What should I do? I threw
them and my candy away. Good and bye! Was it money I was wasting, or just
trash? Don't look back. Look forward. If I could have looked back, I would have
given **"myself"** these suggestions < The name brand of specific items not given at
this time due to intention. >. Go shopping on day one. Buy a supply of items.
My list might have included: five cooked rotisserie chickens, ten cans of tuna
fish, three boxes of hamburger patties, six packages of hot dogs, five jars of
pickles, forty eight low carb drinks, ten low carb energy candy bars, three bags of
emergency low carb jellybeans, three bottles of lemon juice concentrate, two
boxes of artificial sweetener, two bottles of hot sauce, two jars of mustard, six
bottles of seasoning, and several bottles of low carb beer. And while we are
talking about beer, is it polite to be obese and not trying to change? I bring this
up because your condition should help define the desired results of your game.

Do you sip your beer? I don't! I generally turn the bottle up. Why? I want the beer in the bottle to foam. Why? So that the fluid entering into my system has a foaming action. Why? I hope the " fat " and sugar might be washed out of my system with the foaming bubbles. Why? So that my urine might be foamy instead of flat. Why? So that I might be able to see the action of the process at work. Why? So that I might enjoy my effort through the positive reinforcement of seeing the bubbles in the toilet. Why? So that I have to flush the toilet twice. Why? Because the foam won't go down the toilet on the first flush. Amazing, am I saying that I urinated away a one hundred pounds of sugar? Yes and no!

KETOSIS HALITOSIS

In my study of acid and alkaline, I found that asparagus was supposed to have an alkaline affect upon the blood. What I did not know was the effect the asparagus urine was going to have upon the bathroom air. Wow, you can smell it! And I found the same situation with the ketosis concept. Wow, you can smell it. How does it smell? Like fifty year old rotten stale candy. Sometimes I could even see crystals in my urine. Wow, not only can I smell it, but I see it! Yes, and what about your breath? I would suggest that you brush your teeth and use mouthwash several times per day. According to Dr. Atkins' research, the process of ketosis releases fumes < Article: Muscular Development December 2003 Page 80 " No Sex And High Cholesterol For Atkins Diet Spouses". " Atkins dieters also

produce ketones, which gives them breath from hell." " The breath is so bad that
even the man will say, 'Not tonight, dear.' " > < I didn't have to worry about that.
> < I just can't help but tell you a joke: " What comes after celibate? > , which is
"weight" through your breath. And hence, my concern for deep breathing, Out
with the bad air, and in with the good air. So how many beers per day? You see,
the observer may be concentrating on the number of beers, but not me. I am
using a carbohydrate counting and hydraulics theory. Want you call a beer, I call
X number grams of carbohydrate. For example, if I use the twenty grams per day
concept, I ask you, how many of your so called beers can I have? < By the way, I
developed a unique way to count my carbohydrates. I put twenty pennies in a bag.
As the day went along, I would take the number of pennies out of the bag equal to
what I was eating. When I was out of pennies, I was carbohydrate bankrupted for
the day! > Better yet, I am looking at two cans of vegetables. One is a can of
spinach, and the other is a can of green beans. On the back of the cans, under
nutritional facts, they each are said to contain four grams of carbohydrates. But
wait, the four grams is one serving. There are three and one-half servings in each
can! So according to my calculations, each can of what ever is fourteen
carbohydrates in my plan. As I see it, I could eat one can of carbohydrate
vegetables, or drink how many beers at three grams each? You mean they can

send a rocket to Mars, but can't figure out how to solve obesity. Now that is strange! What kind of genius is this?

THEORY OF GENERAL CHANG

Who is General Chang? General Chang is an ultimate supreme leader of the elite force known to the public as Jeds! General Changs style and methods are considered as unorthodox by the council. In the last battle, he was disciplined for breaching the lines of exceptionable format. In the purest sense, he is a warrior! He is the man, to all but himself. This is what makes his ideas and movement so effective. Some say his tactics resemble spiritual, while others say he is crazy or manic. His breath is liken to the dragon, and he plays hard. His philosophy is that when he is coming, he is coming. There is no day after when he comes. Full mental power is his cry, and to suffer is his pleasure. He states that he will spoil your victory with his actions. Just who is General Chang? In the purest sense of the word "war", there are no rules! "All" is fair. Method, means, and motive; all reflect the single objective. To Lose One Hundred Pounds!

HOUSE OF PAIN

We are not the afflicted or the addicted, we are rather the norm; but we pledge to be above average in mind set, to help ourselves to get it going on. We have agreed to not fall by the wayside, although we may be forsaken. We try to smile and laugh, although our bodies may be a aching. For right now a suffering we may be taking. But to become a " Former Fatty Club " member is in our making. So out of my way, and move to the back, the weights coming off as a matter of fact. One day I will say: " How you like me now! "

THE CHAIR EXERCISE CONCEPTS

These are not strength exercises in the traditional sense but multi direction and functional motions and movements designed to help tone, reshape and trim the abdominal area, by which I mean the intestines; and return elasticity to the mid and lower back muscles. These simple movements are the results of using several forms of martial arts and geometrical forms combined with compressing, expanding and stretching also including the dynamic motion sciences. By this I include the arts of Karate, Kung Fu, Tai Chi, Chi Kung, Boxing, Tai boxing, Yoga, Belly Dancing, General Dancing and in specific isometric opening and closing concepts. In consolidating the specific motion concepts, I obtained advice

and consultation from the "Butcher Champions Karate Masters" head instructors.

Different sections of the concept were contributed to by: Grand Master L.R.

Butcher Sr., Sr. Master Edward Butcher Sr., Ki Do Master Edward Butcher Jr.,

Death Master Garcia Davis, and Life Ki Do Master L.R. "Sunny" Butcher Jr., and

in combination with the teachings of The Kicking Ki Do Master "Old Feet of

Flames". All of the concepts were then approved by Grand Master L.R. Butcher,

Sr. In specific, Grand Master Butcher stressed the value of using a holistic

approach to keeping the whole body warm, but to not over tax an already stressed

state, with undue pain, trauma or shock. In addition, Grand Master Butcher

suggested that I seek ways to increase and maintain the thermo output of the body

as a whole unit, rather than to focus upon specific areas. This became part of the

general concept especially in the standing phase of the exercise plan where the

body postures combine free movement with the scientific poses of the physical

arts mentioned earlier, but without the restriction of form kata, or pattern so to

speak. The finial portion of the exercise plan is what is called "Dancing". This

"Dancing" includes free range movement, but retains the general principles of the

previous exercises. And after regular participation one should be ready to rebuild

the muscular strength of the body as needed. In other words, these three steps

should take the participant from the state of "couch potato" to a state called "deconditioned". Then the participant should be ready to increase their muscular abilities unto their desired levels. Look for the upcomming DVD.

THE POSITIVE SIDE OF OBESITY: HAY YOYO

Most times when we hear about people having a body mass index about the suggested value there are only negative comments relating to the topic given. Sure that makes the people in question feel uncomfortable. Here they are being confronted about a situation of which they seem unable to control. In many cases the general idea given for the extra body weight is because the person is either lazy, greedy, or has a medical problem. I now theorize that the answer may be none of the above in many cases. In my opinion, the people who are able to gain large amounts of weight may be of a very specialized order. What I am saying is that there should be a reason why the human body is able to expand to such a large size. What I am doing is taking the so called obesity situation from the realm of being a negative anomaly to that of a positive asset! First I looked to nature to see if I could find an example of an animal that could expand similar to that of humans. After much thought I began to look at the camel. I remembered watching an animal show which explained how before a long trip, say across the desert, the camel would drink a great deal of water. It was said that the camel would store the water in him hump or humps. Oh, some camels have one hump, while other camels have two. With the humps filled with water the camel was ready to start a long trip across the desert. Now for the interesting part, the show explained how the camel would "drink" or use the water from its humps during the trip. Then they showed a camel at the end of the long journey. Guess what? Those water filled humps that once stood on top of the camels back so hard and firm were now sagging off the camel's side. Wow, an animal with its own gas tank and fuel gauge all in one. But then I thought was the increase in humans size because man was suppose to walk for Africa to China? No, to may wild animals I thought. So why might humans have this "obesity ability"? So I began to think about the scriptures. I said to myself that surly there is an answer in there. A short time later, an answer came to me. It was from GENESIS chapter 41 of The Holy Bible sometimes subtitled "Pharaoh's Dreams" where Joseph interpreted the king's dream. Is this proof of knowledge learned from Bible study or what? Then I said "Oh"! Yes, if the king was smart what might he do? Well, I don't know; but if it were me as king I would give the following orders: 1) make storage facilities for all excess food, 2) all food must be removed from it's stalk, 3) everyone must eat as much as they can freely, 4) all that is not eaten must be placed in storage, 5) and nothing at all can be wasted. Basically it would be a seven year party of "eat, drink, and be merry"! Now I ask you, when the famine hits who has the better chance of survival? Is it the "fat" person or the "lean" one? So there you have the core of my obesity theory. I theorize that what is called "obesity" is really part of the human body's specialized survival tools which allows man a great chance of living during times of food shortage. Added to that is what is called the "hunter gatherer" state. In my opinion, man may have originally been a hunter; but if no meat was to be found or man became too weak to hunt efficiently, then man could still survive by consuming gathered items. Now if the human system burns meats as fuel, but stores fuel from gathered products, then this would imply that the human system already anticipates the food supply situations man has experienced. Of course this is before the invention of: 1) the supermarket, 2) canning, 3) bottling 4) freezing and 5) the freezer itself. We need to remember that man is living in a modified environment to say the least. In addition, man now has the ability to mix different foods from all around the world at one sitting. This also is a part of mans modified environment. Once upon a time, long long ago, man could only eat what was native to the area he was in. I ask you, one thousand years ago, how could you get an ice cream cone from the North Pole to Africa? Figure that out! My conclusion is that in a large number of cases that the state called obesity is coming from a lack of knowledge about how the human body works. I also theorize that the condition call diabetes is an effort of the human system to stop the conversion of food into stored energy called fat. It is my opinion based upon the information that I have gathered the state called diabetes occurs in two ways depending upon the fat storage type of body a person has. If we return to our camel examples, we can see in theory how a double hump camel could retain more water than a single hump camel. If we apply this type of thinking to the human body, we can derive two conclusions. One type of body stores only a limited amount of fat before insulin production and fat conversion is disrupted chemically resulting in diabetes. The second type of body type may expand greatly storing vast amounts of energy in the form of fat before insulin production and fat conversion is disrupted chemically resulting in diabetes. I now theorize that the state called diabetes in both body types is a result of a stored fat maximum condition. The question may be in many cases just how much fuel as fat can your gas tank < which is the body > store. This theory would also explain what is called the "yo-yo" effect that some dieters have experienced. If my feast or famine theory is correct, than to "yo-yo" in weight would be a natural function of the body. A simple response to the food intake quantity, quality, and variations in combination.

BIBLICIAL EXAMPLE: PHARAOH'S DREAM

THE HOLY BIBLE: NEW LIVING TRANSLATION: ISBN: 0-8423-4050-5
GENESIS 41: 14-38

Pharaoh sent for Joseph at once, and he was brought hastily from the dungeon. After a quick shave and change of clothes, he went in and stood in Pharaoh's presence. I had a dream last night," Pharaoh told him, "and none of these men can tell me what it means. But I have heard that you can interpret dreams, and that is why I have called for you."

It is beyond my power to do this," Joseph replied, But God will tell you what it means and and will set you at ease."

So Pharaoh told him the dream. "I was standing on the bank of the Nile River," he said. "Suddenly, seven fat, healthy-looking cows came up out of the river and began grazing along its bank. But then seven other cows came up from the river. They were very thin and gaunt- in fact, I've never seen such ugly animals in all the land of Egypt. These thin, ugly cows ate up the seven fat ones that had come out of the river first; but afterward they were still as ugly and gaunt as before! Then I woke up.

A little later I had another dream. This time there were seven heads of grain on one stalk, and all seven heads were plump and full. Then out of the same stalk came seven withered heads, shriveled by the east wind. And the withered heads swallowed up the plump ones! I told these dreams to my magicians, but not one of them could tell me what they mean."

"Both dreams mean the same thing," Joseph told Pharaoh. "God was telling you what he is about to do. The seven fat cows and the seven plump heads of grain both represent seven years of prosperity. The seven thin, ugly cows and the seven withered heads of grain represent seven years of famine. This will happen just as I have described it, for God has shown you what he is about to do. The next seven years will be a period of great prosperity throughout the land of Egypt. But afterward there will be seven years of famine so great that all the prosperity will be forgotten and wiped out. Famine will destroy the land. This famine will be so terrible that even the memory of the good years will be erased. As for having the dream twice, it means that the matter has been decreed by God and that he will make these events happen soon.

"My suggestion is that you find the wisest man in Egypt and put him in charge of a nationwide program. Let Pharaoh appoint officials over the land, and let them collect one-fifth of all the crops during the seven good years. Have them gather all the food and grain of these good years into the royal storehouses, and store it away so there will be food in the cities. That way there will be enough to eat when the seven years of famine come. Otherwise disaster will surely strike the land, and all the people will die."

Joseph Made Ruler of Egypt

Joseph's suggestions were well received by Pharaoh and his advisers. As they discussed who should be appointed for the job, Pharaoh said, "Who could do it better than Joseph? For he is a man who is obviously filled with the spirit of God."

BEST FRIEND SCALE

July 20, 2005 update.

I have suddenly realized that there are two very important tools you may need when regulating ones intake in this manner. The first key to this diet plan is the twenty pennies and a plastic bag. The second major to is "the bathroom scale." The scale must become your friend. Now once you reach your goal weight, you might want to drop down an extra five pounds. The reason for this is to give you yo-yo room. Now place a big piece of tape on the scale where you can write yu weight upon it. What I mean is your ideal weight before yu take off the additional five pounds. Now remember you have given yourself five pounds of "play room." So when the scale reaches yur desired weight number, you know it's time to return to your twenty pennies. This way you can take action before you notice it in kyur camel humps sometimes called love handles. You just have to watch that sneeky fat conversion. "A scale a day helps keep the camel fat bags away!"

AFTERWORD

AUTHORS UPDATE

< This is hot, this is hot, fresh, it's very fresh. The Chang is going hot, the core is over flooding. The Chang has gone hot, the core is on fire! 8/02/05 > I don't really want to start any new chapters because the book is basically done, but.

HOW I CAUGHT THE BUFFALO

Anyway, I had left Egypt after spending many years there. So I was walking across North America when suddenly a fellow of one eighth full Indian blood sprang out upon me. There he was a seven eighths naked one eighth full blood North American Indian. Bow, arrow, bushy hair and all. Then he said to me: "Me huntum famous buffalo. Me seeum you and say "there is famous buffalo". Then I comeum upon you only to find you not famous buffalo at all; but you beum famous buffalo butt! How didum get da buffalo butt?" Man step off. I have not idea what you are talking about. So after my meeting with the one

eighth full blood North American Indian, I continued my journey to China. It

took a while but I made it. I had walked all the way from Egypt to China; ahhh, I

did not walk across the water. I hear someone else did that. Anyway, when I

arrived in China a great number of people were happy to greet me.   As I began

to walk down The Great Walkway the crowd began to shout; "Fu Lu Boo Fulu,

Boofulu, Boofulu, Boofulu Boo Fulu Boofulu! As I walked up the temple steps

they shouted the same. Fu Lu Boo Fulu, Boofulu, Boofulu, Boofulu Boo Fulu

Boofulu! This shouting lasted until the very second that I sat in the royal chair at

"The Table of Boo Fu Lu!" Then the great leader, Master Chang, came into the

room. He bowed as he entered and when he came to "The Table of Boo Fu Lu"

Master Chang took a seat at the table and asked if I had any questions. Yes, yes I

do have a question I replied. "Why do you bow when you enter a room?" "Aw,

you seek knowledge. Master Chang can help you. Long ago, the ancient decided

to help the people. He noticed how weak and brittle the people had become. It is

written that a great number were found with at Boo Fulu. Word was sent to

Egypt, but with at Boo Fulu was there too. And so, in Egypt they began to write

high upon the walls. This was two fold. Knowledge was everywhere, and it

helped the stiff neck people with their stiff necks. In China our leader told us to

look at the tree tops, the mountains tops, the stars directly over your head, and the ceilings. I hear in other parts of the world < Rome > they began to paint upon the

ceilings. Yes, ahhh, yes; this was a part of an ancient healing science. You have

come to Master Chang. Another leader decided to make bowing an everyday part

of the culture. So he made an edict that when a person walked into a room, the

person would bow; and when two people would greet; the two would bow to each

other. Now due to the martial arts this was tricky. So it was written that the

younger of the two of the same sex would bow first; but in the martial aspect the

lesser rank would bow first and stay as such until acknowledged by the rank.

Now if two students have the same rank, they could bow as they pleased. Ahhh,

you want to know why from Master Chang? Ahhh, because, if they bow at the

same time and crack each other in the head; ahhh, the same ranks always bump

heads, especially at tournament! Ah ha! I am Master Chang. But the origin of

this comes from thee ancient desire to keep the peoples back supple and stomach

coiled and elastic. Yes, yes, yes; what you call Karate is really Karate Do

pronounced < Doe >. Thee martial arts were originally developed for the famed

Tin Man. The arts were designed to keep his joints lubricated and in alignment.

The books of wisdom were written for the Scarecrow who was so dumb that he

thought he was without brain. Let Master Chang tell you my son, all three were

in terrible shape when they came to Chi Na. All three had been cast out of Egypt.

Yes, yes yes! Each had their own problem. It had rained upon The Tin Man while he was sitting. He rusted like the Scarecrow on fire, so they put him in a wheeled chair and he road it around behind the stinky animals. They called it chair Ra rot < chariot >. He had come to learn the forms, which are postures so the oils could penetrate his joints. He was all rusty, but, after doing the regeneration forms or postures, he was like the rising morning sun < Ra >. And so, they called him C-3-PO. Now "O" being the fourth vowel my friend, in a certain language, my son, meant the number four. So, the cipher of his name is 3-3-6 to the second power and four which is daleth in hidden form. Daleth in a certain science was said to be able to move up and down the central shaft of the mystical tree. This implied the regeneration form. But he also was very ignorant when he came to Chi Na. Now and so, the teacher said he was a very ignorant man being when he came. Originally he was known as C-3-P which ciphered into 3-3-6 of the second level, or 666/666. And hence he had the mental markings of beast and man. They say he was very important. Setting himself upon the fire, lo, made of straw. In Egypt they were going to make him into a brick, but lo, his head was too hard. They say it was as brick but not stone or rock. Now once he obtained the lessons, he received the letter of the mystical Egyptian "O" unto his name. Then his name is ciphered, metaphysically speaking, as 3-3-6-4. The two threes imply a hidden Alpha or 1. And so it was discovered that his name had reflected his birthday which contained the numbers 1, 3, 6, and 4. Then they added the numbers together and found 3+3+6+4=16 and 1+3+6+4=14. Now the 1+6=7 which implied the highest level in a certain science; while the 1+4=5 which implied the flesh or while in the flesh. Hum, I am Master Chang. Now the final clue came when the hermeneutics calculated 16+14, or PN. This was his mystic number. In the cipher, PN is his mystic code number. 64. That is what he had to beat. And so, he was born before that. Now, PN= 6+4=FD but because his is 16&14 an alpha or double Alpha is implied. Did you see the television series "Numbers" my son, or have you ever heard the mystic musical jam by "Wayne The Great" DJ from O'Dell's < who demonstrated Transcendental Music Evocation Meditation > pump the song "Numbers" by the group Kraftwork!? Ahhh ha, let Master Chang tell you my son, 1+6 is 7, 1+4 is 5, 7+5 is 12, and 1+2=3. 3 is the number of vision. The letter C. See! 16+14=P+N=PIN, I being an Alpha raised to the second power and so is hidden. 16+14=30. Now the thirteenth letter of a twenty six letter alpha beta is daleth raised to the second power of which is capital daleth. Daleth in cipher form is the dale spelled DalEth. The E being the physical five pointed star which represents symbolically the human body. Once the body is moving along the path towards the goal of the will of ones mental mind intention, one is said to be upon The Dial or ROTA as in tarot or Torah. The pure willed ability to move up and down the mystical tree of the central path in a certian science. And so, he was awarded the mystical level of 30 or C squared, or six, which is an F by the famed Butchers Family of Butchers Champions Karate Masters here in Chi Na. It is said that he had learned several arts including the famed Grand Masters snapping brick technique, but he teaches no one, no one except his students. Who are they? Hum? Now to the. Stop my son, You are confused, or so it is written. The three are as one. So you can see, how the Tin Man and the Scarecrow Man are connected. The Yellow Bricked Road is the mystical path to enlightenment, my son. All want to see the Wee Zard. Wee being more than one, and Zard being XYZ from the back of RA, being Able, movable Daleth of whom is generally located behind the scenes or certain. Now, Scarecrow ciphers into $9 < I$ = alpha or second power alpha, which would be Alpha or S? ScareCrow = SC = $9/3$ = 27 = $26 + 1$ = LARGE ALPHA, $2 + 7 = 9$, which is I. I is the lessor of S which both are of a 9 basic root. And 3, which is C, is also the squared root of 9. $9+3=12$. 12 is the number of the zodiac. But, there is more than one zodiac. There is the lesser zodiac of The Earths Sun and The Greater Zodiac about the cosmic galactic core And so, there is 12 in 12 or 144 houses of The Great Zodiac. But $1+4+4=9$, so what is the tenth level? The opening of the cosmic way; the mystic 13 house of the zodiac. The cosmic alignment. To see the core. We are almost done my friend. You see, Da Grand Master would tell his student that "Naaaa Naaaa na, it went down just as I had planned it, pluaaaaaa < the sound of a horse at rest, crazy horse says the

Sr. Master >." Now unto The Cowardly Lion, ahhh we in Chi Na call him The

Sissy < lion >. Let Master Chang explain. It is said that The Lion was kicked out

of Egypt after being taught by our brothers "The Hidden In Plain View Egyptian

Masters" because of domestication. Yes, he had become very familiar. More like

a human rather than a lion. He was very friendly. Everyone loved him, that is

until he read a certain book from cover to cover. A book of vision < see: "They

Live", the movie > and so he became very fearful of this and of that. Almost

starving to death, he lost it all. All of it, why not take all of it; and so the song

went < by Bootsy >! With a certain book in hand, in the face of The Sphinx, a

swift kick to goraf < Go-RA-F: "Beyond The Thunder Dome", the movie > and

so he came with yall. You, You, You and Boo-FuLu You too. And so, it is

written, The ancient Masters of "Butchers" took pity and mercy upon him, The

Sissy! And they taught him, The Sissy. Scare of The Sphinx, half man head, half

lion body of Egypt! And so, he, The Sissy, was sent to Shiolin for the animal

training forms and to school for his addiction unto that woman called Dorothy,

The Scorpion whose sting is said to be worse that Death itself. And so, he The

Sissy, learned from Master Splinter himself < Movie: "Teenage Mutant Ninja

Turtles" > and Master YodDa < YodDa=Yod which is hand and Da which

implies motion-upon the mystic tree of the zodiac of whom Yoda is The Bunny

rabi T of the East Tear curtain, a tear being to cry out from the prison of the flesh

>. And so, The Sissy lion learned the animal forms: the rat, the rabbit, the Aunt

T's tiger, and so on. What was wrong? Oh, the domesticated lions roar is raaaah,

but the wild lion says woooohooo! So, the Sissy Lion could not speak the word,

or was difficult of speech. Sounds familiar. So, he, the Sissy Lion learned the

zodiac forms of She Lion < Shaolin > to ready himself to meet the female animal

of the scorpion style called The Black Widow. And so she came, but and so he

escaped her evil vile wicked devouring black widow spider triune grasping fist

form < and the people said; "Go Sissy, go, go Sissy" >. It is also said that The

Sissy had learned the style of them whom guard the mystic door, The Apes < See:

Planet Of The Apes I, II, III, IV, the new Planet Of The Apes, Congo, > Well to

be exact see: The Mask, Shogan Assassin I, II, III and IV, Zaram, The X Men I/II,

Sin City, The Keep, Doctor Detroit, Man On Fire, Fallen, The Fifth Element,

Enter The Dragon, The Game of Death 25th anniversary Edition, Death Race

2000, Isla She Wolf Of The S. S. I&II, Terminator I/II/III, Matrix I/II/III, Bootsy

in concert 1978, Star Trek I/II/III/IV, all Bat Man's movies, Ultra Man, Predator

I/II/III, all The Alien movies, The Order, Death Wish I/II/III/IV, The

Exterminator, The Mac, Come Home Charleston Blue, The Blues Brothers I/II,

Remo Williams I/II, Total Recall, The Nerds, Lord Of Illusions, Pulp Fiction,

Unbreakable, The Cube I/II of which are high level science, Indian Jones I/II/III,

The Golden Child, Harlem Nights, Raw, Richard Pryor, all James Bond movies,

The Invisible Man, My Way, Contact, and When We Were Kings. Now once

The Sissy Lion had learned the skills, he had to be taught the mental discipline

due to his affliction. His affliction was he loved Dorothy. He did not realize that

he was an animal. It is said that Master Meta 3.14 taught The Sissy the famous

1,000 Strokes Of The Chinnabar Kundalini Sexual Tantra Set. So, as I, Master

Chang, has explained the answer unto you; I, Master Chang, have a question of

my own. Ahh, yes ahh, how did shu < you > caught Boo-Fu-Lu?" What? What

Boo-Fu-Lu? "Ha, you have Boo-Fu-Lu!" I didn't have any idea what Master

Chang was talking about? What is this Boo-Fu-Lu anyway? Then Master Chang

pointed and smiled while saying "Boo-Fu-Lu!" What! Boo-Fu-Lu, Buffalo? I

then asked if he was saying Buffalo? He replied: "Yaa, ahhh, Bok Men." What?

I know he is not calling me Buffalo Butt Bookman from the television series

Goodtimes. Do you mean Buffalo Butt Bookman? Haa, yes it's you.

BOO-FU-LU

  So how did I catch the mystical Boo-Fu-Lu or Buffalo Butt Bookman affliction?

Oh it was easy. I became overweight due to reading, studying, and writing these

books.

FRANK M. CONAWAY, JR.

HOUSE OF KI DO

In the martial arts style of The Baltimore Maryland Butcher's Family there are many styles. These styles comprise what is called "The House Of Ki Do." Now as far as styles are concerned, this topic was discussed by Bruce Lee at great length. I found his verbal explanation to be very hard to comprehend. In addition, when I had begun training in the Death Ki Do system, I found that each of The Masters were similar in general, but very different in specific. In other words you could tell that each of them was of similar origin; but each of them were vastly different. In a way they were each roses; but each had different colored petals. This seemed very strange indeed. How could this be? It was because of "styles". You see, it is easy for a man who has been trained or disciplined in many forms or styles to say he believes in none of them; but it makes no sense what so ever for the man whom knows no style to make the same comment. What is being stated is relative to the level the martial student is upon. Sure there is no one way a person is suppose to be, but every person starts out as human. And although every person starts out as human, once their character unfolds, each will be, act, and react as a uniquely different individual. The same is true for styles. If we examine Shiolin Temple, we might call all the students by the same tile. But once we understand that Shiolin Temple Boxing was divided into subjects and levels, we can begin to see how a style can be no style. Each form within Shiolin has its own fundamentals or basics. When I say form, I mean like Snake or Tiger style. Now once the student learned the basics of a form or style, such as in snake fist; they would move on to another form or style such as Tiger Claw or Fist. Now these were called the animal forms. In general, each student would stay in a class for a style or form until the basics were learned. Once the basics were learned, they would move on to another style. These styles or animal form sets were called chambers. One might say The Snake Fist Form Chamber, and so on. Now once the student rotates to each chamber; they were considered to have learned all the basics of The Animal Forms. Now it was time for the student to graduate. At this point it should be noted that each of the students "style" appeared basically the same. This is a general statement. Now graduation could mean one of two things. It would all be a matter of choice. Does the student want to return to one of the animal chambers to master that animal form, or does the student want to go on to learn other skills such as a weapon style. Then there are other things such as: Fa Jing, Point Striking, Chi Kung, Yin Tai Chi, Yang Tai Chi, Tai Chi Twan, etc. Now as you add these different skills to the basic student's style, the appearance of the techniques seem to change. Now once the student has mastered enough styles, he then becomes as one with certain parts of the many forms of his knowledge. This incorporation of techniques and ideas into ones life causes the student to become unique to his

gathered body of knowledge. And hence, the student of many styles has become

a style of styles without there being a style. He and his style are one. He is his

style of no style at all. A very unique blend suited for himself. No such style at

all. This is called "to become!" In The House Of Ki Do, the same type of

situation exists. Only here it is really not seen, nor very rarely talked about. But

what I can say is that among the Ki Do styles in The House Of Ki Do, there is

Death Ki Do, and Spiritual Ki Do. Now as far as external styles are concerned, I

can say that it has been said that Death Ki Do is "a style of all styles." That's not

to say that all styles are included in the martial knowledge of Death Ki Do; but it

certainly does not imply that any are excluded from inclusion!

HARD KNOWLEDGE

What was the hardest part of the learning that I gained? No, it was not

putting it into practice. Nor was it all of the hard reading of books. The second

hardest part was to try to understand "what I" understood in a way that I could tell

others who had no idea what I was talking about, the new information that I had

learned. The hardest part was when I realized that I needed to tell others what I

found by writing the information and emotions. The worst of it was knowing what I had comprehended in my own mind. The battle cry became: "I must finish my work!" It seemed very simple to me. Anyone who wanted to help me would help me "finish my work!" Ninety something plus times this did not happen. Instead, the non verbal response was to do anything but help me finish my work. Rap, talks, questions, rebuttals, comparisons and all of The Reasons why not. This was the terrible burden of the whole task. Even unto them whom had nothing better to do than "try" to attack my mind with their own mental confusion. Yes, people can pass on negative vibrations to another person. Yes, people can cause negative vibrations to exist in others environments. Yes, this to is a form of peer pressure. And how might you perceive the affects of that negative pressure. At this point, I believe the working force might mimic a form of Traumatic Stress Syndrome. When I say Traumatic Stress Syndrome, I mean the stress levels that approach the maximum value of the physical side of the negative encounters can handle. In most cases, there will be a maximum or full load point. This is the greatest point of stress of the whole situation. Now that is a physical challenge. But, when the physical challengers also attempt to break ones drive or spirit, quite often the attack is going to extend into the mind. You must realize that a physical situation most times can be somewhat repaired, but when the mind is over taxed; who knows what can be done in the unseen world. And so, here also is a great work. When the mind comes under attack from the ego of others, one may be placed in a situation that would ordinarily cause ones

mind to snap. The physical results of ones mind snapping could be expressed in

millions of way. Some are known to doctors, and some are not. But in The

House of the Phionx, there is another way. This has to do with the martial skill.

In the martial arts, when one comes under great attack, one must be able to focus

upon the objective. This ability is known as being able to "Lock!" Locking in a

combat situation implies being able the defend and attack while being under what

is called "in coming!"

METAPHYSICAL MOVIE CIPHERS PREVIEW

Predator 3: The Kundalini Hermenentic Metaphysical Movie Cipher

INTRODUCTION ONLY

What is Kundalini? In short, the science of Kundalini deals with an ancient

science that shows certain people how to balance their electromagnetic centers

called in one system chakras. Hermeneutics deals with a specialized form of

biblical or scripture interpretation. The question should be asked as to why the

scriptures might need to interpreted. First of all, much of the book called The

Holy Bible is written in one of four general cipher forms: parables, mysteries, wonders, and sealed. Second due to the general time of the last "official" writing date to today, there is a large gap in "the transition" or motion that is affecting what is called "spiritual knowledge" or "spiritual historical lineage". Metaphysics deals with what is called "a science form" above physics. I understand these words but what do these words mean when placed together? In general, the laws of the science called physics remain the same and cannot be broken. This form of theory science is called Physics. The rules and principles of Physics come under what is called "The Theory of Relativity". The main governing principle of The Theory of Relativity is: "nothing moves faster than the speed of Light!" Now, when we turn to the theories of Metaphysic, one could look at the theories of "Specific Relativity!" Why? Because Specific Relativity says;" sure there are things that move faster than the speed of Light!" So at this point I should say that ancient Metaphysical theories deal with cosmic zodiac energy induction, multi dimensional movement, internal exploration of the human mind, and/or more. What do I mean by Kundalini Hermeneutic Metaphysical Movie Cipher? I will use my knowledge of these various sciences to try to explain what is being relayed to the movie audience upon another level. On a level that may be seen but not known. Knowledge!

Tuesday June 28, 2005, I had often thought about this movie; but I just could not make "a sense" about it. I was thinking about the movie during a severe rain storm. There was nothing do. Why? Because of the great deal of

thunder and lightening. So, I began to think about the Predators face when he

took off his helmet. Kundalini Objective: what is the general objective of the

Kundalini Science? It should be said that knowledge is knowledge, but

knowledge is of value upon what the one with the knowledge intends to do with

it! There are several answers to this question, of which I would like to provide a

few: to know, to see or watch, to control, to become one with, and become. To

know has to do with being intelligent in the theories of the general topic. To see

has to do with being able to observe the motion or manifestation of the general

sciences upon the physical plane. To control has tot due with acquiring special

abilities where as one can affect "the reality" by mind intention. To become one

with generally implies to become a master or living channel of some form of

element or entity of what is called creation. This concept of creation generally

implies becoming a lesser element. To become implies what is unfoldment. This

unfoldment generally refers to moving towards a specific goal or designed place

of choice. Now let's see if we can find examples of these concepts. An example

of to know is sometimes known as Oricial. If you look at the Matrix movies, you

see how the Oricial gave interpretation by questioning the character Neo. This

form of interaction is called to show the ways, but not to influence the character.

An example of "to see" can be seen in the Predator Two movie. Notice how the seer or watcher threw "the bones", which is a form of what is called the science of divination. Notice what The Seer said to Danny Glover: "How can you stop what can't be stopped?" On the level of to control, we generally have three levels of controllers. It should be said that the controllers are generally involved in the process.

LAST NOTES

Each of these concepts has a story behind them. Maybe I will write about them some other time. Right now I want to give you a few more things to think about. Increase your breathing. Try to draw more air into your body. Expand your chest like the red breasted Robin. Instead of breathing in then out, try to breathe in longer. You might want to count your breathes. One to one, two to one, three to one and so on.

1) Practice what Grand Master L.R. Butcher called coiling. This means to lightly bounce your upper body upon your stomach muscles. You also want to draw your stomach muscles in tightly and hold them. You can do this at your desk, while you drive, on the subway or bus. As you breathe in lift your chest upward. Roll your shoulders back. Now with you stomach

already tight and sucked in, exhale by pushing the stomach muscles further. Wow, can you feel it?

2) Try to work on your posture. Why do children generally have better posture than adults? The world is new to them so they look up often. Adults are taller than them, and so again they must look upward to speak face to face. Look at the clouds above your head. Look at the tree tops. Look at the ceiling. Does it need to be painted? Why do you think some ceilings have designs on them anyway? Hold your chin up and stick out your chest. Oh, by the way, yes people are going to think you are crazy. So what!

3) I would like to note that the martial arts are full of postures and poses that help keep the human body in order. The element of violence is not the real focus of the martial arts. When a person practices alone there is no one to fight.

4) Squeeze your buttocks muscles. Tighten up on that loose booty or do the rump shaker.

5) Remember to never become hungry. If you do, you might look for the quickest source of fuel-sugar!

6) Remember to be positive. Take control. Help yourself.

JACKING META

One day I was having a discussion with a friend about my e-book concept. My friend asked me a very serious question. "Don't you worry that people will just copy your work and give it to their friends?" "What do you mean?" I replied. "Don't you think people might jack you, house you, clip you, dub and remix you, Audi 500 you, get low on you, smooth Willy you, do the bird on you, 52 pick up you, back door you, cyber funk you, bootleg you, or Cutty on parole cause Cutty has to roll you?" Yes and sure. "Yes people might due such a thing" I replied. You must remember that obesity is being in a state or emergency. In a state of emergency all the rules sometimes may have to be broken. How can people think clearly while they are under the affliction? People need help, and they need it NOW! But I believe the average person is fair. I especially believe that if my work helps someone, they one day will remember me. They will know that my work is my love for humanity. They will be able to see that after I healed myself I didn't forget them. Writing this book was hard. Some people critize me for my writing style, grammar, or use of less than/greater than signs for brackets. Let me tell you something, I remember the people who helped me, and I remember those who didn't. I remember those who said you can do it, and I remember those < of whom I have proven wrong, apology not excepted at all, na, not, and none > who said I was crazy or there abouts. Maybe a person may feel that they have to try the concepts first before they buy a copy of my work. Maybe a person might have to reach their objective before they remember me. Either way, I believe that if I really help a person they will some how return the favor. They will know. But most importantly of all, "I Know". I know that some how, in between the time I was born unto today, I had gained the capacity to extend love, my love into the world. I would like to thank the world for providing me with this opportunity. In Egypt it is written: "Man Heal Thy Self." I came, I saw, I conquered- Northwestern Class of 1980 The Wild Cats! Howard University School of Architecture starting date 1980. The Champions/ Butchers Champions Karate Masters- "It's time to go home!" To Booty and Nubia- "at the metaphysical gates ya'll!" To LL, Kel L, Funk O, and 05/21/05 Jah Mi El / The day I first knew of you, but I had seen you in my dreams / Read "Thee Book" FROM COVER TO COVER IN ORDER and See. Love Meta Pop Pop! P.S. That's an order form the council. Be wise, use knowledge. The fool often speaks against that which they know not. The wise man knows it's subject to bite them in the ass-ets. Some say that experience is the best teacher. I don't know about that, but I can say it is very convincing. Answer that of Revelations 13:18 and you will know something. I love you boy. "A man has to do what a man has to do!" Why? Because, they won't < and didn't >! Meta Out.

HELP ME META

I understand that what you are reading might not make sense to you. I understand that you might still have questions. Look how long it took me to understand what I knew for my self. No, start today, you will understand. But if you still have questions first refer to my other books " Proof Of Ketosis and What Can I Eat ", then you can ask me your questions by sending me your email to " askmeta " at hotmail.com.. The way this works is that you can ask me up to five questions. I will answer up to three questions if I can. Then I will post your ansers with the questions and your email account, name, or code name at " lulu.com/meta314 ". Please give me about 30 days, but chek back and I should have it posted. There will be a small download cost for your special questions. You have to pay the download price before you get the answers that I have given. If I can't answer your questions, then I will send you an free response email that I don't have the knowledge of your questions. I thank you, and I am trying to show my love for you. You can do it, I know this because I did.

FRANK M. CONAWAY, JR.

THE LAST DROP

Its strange, was thinking about some of the information I had read from the medical documents so I decided to go on the internet to view the lions statistics. Next I decided to compare his weight to his meat and water consumption. Then I compared his statistics to the suggested six foot man with proper body mass index. Oh, now I see; but then something very very strange happened. I had a thought. Then I began to laugh. Wow, so I found that diets that invoked ketosis were called ketogenic diets. Now a diet is defined as: < Diet: the food and drink that a person, animal, or group usually takes; customary nourishment, the kind and amount of food selected for a person or animal for specific reason (as ill health or obesity) (a high-protein diet), something provided specially habitually (as for enjoyment) (a steady diet of television) Merriam-Webster's High School Dictionary 1996 ISBN 0-03-096484-9 Page 247 >. So if I were observing a carnivorous animals eating habits, what would I say about it. Suppose an animal, say a lion, became domesticated and suddenly found himself obese, could my diet plan help him. I think so. But I have never seen a lion count pennies. What other name or title could I give my work so that the obese carnivores by nature, but now domesticated carbohydrate eating herbivore could understand the concepts?

Then I asked myself as to why might the other authors that knew about the ketoses process did not use the term in their diets title? Hum, why? Well if they won't I will. So this diet plans technical name is: The Low < Low Carbohydrate > Ketosis Hydration Thermal Intestine Ketogenic Diet Plan. Its trade name is " The 20 Pennies A Day Diet Plan". Then I knew it was complete when I thought of Egypt. So this is "The 20 Pennies A Day Diet Plan", also known as: 1) The Carbohydrates You Eat Turn To Sugar Diet Plan, 2) The That's Not Fat It's Liquid Carbohydrate Sugars Diet Plan, 3) The Eat Like A Lion Diet Plan, 4) The Meat And Water Diet Plan, 5) The Carnivores Diet Plan, 6) The Ketosis Diet Plan, 7) The Conaway Jr. Diet Plan, 8) The Hotep Is Knowledge Diet Plan, 9) The Low Carb Beer Diet Plan, 10) The Chug That Beer Diet Plan, 11) The Our Daily Meat Diet Plan, 12) The Let The Adults Eat Meat Diet Plan, 13) The North Pole Diet Plan, 14) The Omnivorous Ways Of Eating Diet Plan, 15) The Eating For Insulin Verses Gluagon Diet Plan, 16) The Zero Carb Approach Diet Plan, 17) The Eat Like A Polar Bear Diet Plan, 18) The Royal Ravens Changing Of The Guards Diet Plan, and 19) The Egyptian Sphinx Diet Plan. Head of a man, body of a lion. Then I began to really laugh. Why? Because if any of these titles that I have named are not in use, then they all belong to me! Ah Ha.

FRANK M. CONAWAY, JR.

GOURMAND: EATING FOR A PLEASURE PRINCIPLE

I now realize that along with not understand how the human system works,
made may have also increased his own will or desire to " overeat " by learning
how to please the tongue and taste buds. I theorize that the art of cooking could
also be fueling the obesity epidemic. Looking at my model the lion, I realize that
he kills and eats for survival. I find that in general man has developed a
psychological attitude that he wants his food to taste certain ways so that he can
derive pleasure from the taste of what he is eating. In reality, the true taste of the
food may be masked by seasons and other preparation steps such as breading.
Then also we must consider the usage of broth and gravy. Think about it. Why do
you add butter and salt to greens. Why do you add butter, sugar, and spices to
baked sweet potatoes. I think they describe cooking something as it is as being
"bland". So the addition of these exotic flavors to the basic food " is an effort to
do what? How about make the consumption process " enjoyable ". A gourmand is
described as one who is excessively fond of eating and drinking, a person heartily
interested in good food and drink. A gourmet is described as a connoisseur of
food and drink. A connoisseur is described as a person qualified to act as a judge
in matters involving taste and appreciation. Addition is described as the quality or

state of being addicted, compulsory physical need for a habit-forming drug <

Merriam Webster's HIGH SCHOOL DICTIONARY ISBN 0-03-096484-9 >.

The question now becomes how often are you eating to please you mouth?

And I should add The Bible even speaks of something that is sweet to the lips but

bitter to the stomach < Revelation 10:10 >. I would also like to note that "

animals raised in captivity do not, as a rule, have the skills to survive in the wild"

< LIFE: America's Weekend Magazine August 05, 2005 page 12 >.

Behaviourism: "The central tenet of behaviourism is that thoughts, feelings, and

intentions, mental processes all, do not determine what we do. Our behaviour is

the product of our conditioning. We are biological machines and do not

consciously act; rather we react to stimuli. <THE OXFORD COMPANION TO

THE MIND Edited by Richard L. Gregory ISBN 0-19-866124-X page 71>"

Smell: " In vertebrates we define smell as involving the stimulation of the first

cranial nerve, the olfactory nerve. < page 720 >" Taste: "Flavour is usually

defined as the overall sensation of taste and smell. Taste refers to sensations

arising from the taste receptors in the mouth and throat while smell arises from

receptors in the nose. < page 767 >" Thinkers, Independent: On the whole, Homo

sapiens tends to be conventional: that is, very few people have revolutionary

ideas. At an early age, for instance, virtually every child is taught that the earth is

a globe, revolving round the sun in a period of one year-and he or she will believe it. Yet a mere six hundred years ago, children who were taught at all learned that the sun goes round the earth, and they believed that with equal fervour. Consider, for instance, the Flat Earthers. The belief in a world shaped like a pancake is very old, but the fact that it lingers on is strange. < page 772 >" Addiction: For most people the concept of drug addition is dominated by images of physical and mental degradation brought by the use of heroin and cocaine. It is generally forgotten that the most widely used drugs are caffeine in tea and coffee, nicotine, and alcohol; and that the most successful drug pushers are tobacconists and publicans. Of course the great majority of those who enjoy these drugs are not necessarily addicted, if addicted means a tendency to excessive use of the drug, a craving for it when it is not available, and the development of a variety of physical and psychological symptoms when it is suddenly withdrawn. Addiction is a difficult word to define and a WHO expert committee in 1970 substituted the words 'drug dependence'. This is characterized by psychological symptoms such as craving and a compulsion to take the drug on a continuous or periodic basis, and physical effects developing when the drug is withheld or is unavailable. < page 3-4 >" Abnormal: " describes behavior or an event that differs from the familiar or usual. Just how bizarre, unusual, or even antisocial behavior must be in order to be classified as 'abnormal' depends on many factors that change with **knowledge** and with social perceptions. Thus, for example, classification might depend upon whether or not the behavior was socially acceptable or whether there were symptoms, however minor, or an underlying problem or disease already regarded as abnormal. Such classification is helpful when it leads to useful treatment, therapy, or special education, but it can also be dangerous, for in extreme cases it can take an unusual or gifted person away from society. The probability of an abnormal event occurring against chance can be predicted from statistical tests. In scientific research such tests are important in establishing whether an event is unusual enough to require special explanation. In clinical situations, however, applicable tests are difficult to establish, because classifications of abnormal events depend on factors that are changeable. < page 1 >" Accident Proneness: " is a deceptively easy term. We all know what it means but we do not all mean the same thing. Since the ambiguities arise partially because of the way we speak about accidents, it may be helpful to clarify this term. An accident refers to the results of an action, generally to an unplanned, even an unexpected result. It has been described as an event with said consequences, but the relationship between the proceeding behaviour and the consequences is not at all simple. A time-honored example of an accident is a person falling flat as he slips on a banana-skin--an act, incidentally, that few have ever witnessed and which conveys the impression that the world at one time must have been littered with banana-skins. In such an example the person who slips has the accident for which he was partly responsible. But we also speak of someone

having an accident when something falls on him. A spills a cup of tea over B and

we say that B has suffered an accident. To add to the confusion, different kinds of

action result in similar accidents, while the same act often has very different

results. Hence, if we are to understand accidents we need to understand the

proceeding behavior. But accident data are usually only records of the outcome of

actions.

In 1971 Shaw published her comprehensive analysis of accident proneness. She

avoided an extreme position. She concluded that many characteristics of behavior

change with age and that it is not true that most accidents are sustained but a

small number of people. But she examined in detail earlier studies and

demonstrated the importance of certain factors such as 'attention (defined as the

ability to choose quickly and perform a corrective response to a sudden stimulus),

the stability of behaviour, and the involuntary control over motor behaviour. She

supported the study of car drivers-' a man drives as he lives'-and the finding that

a bad civil record tends to indicate a bad accident risk. < page 1-2 >"

CHUG BEERS

First I would like to explain why I have two books that are very similar in text. Due to the topic and the open action of them whom would be called critics, I find it necessary to approach the desired audience from two directions. Now group one may be against beer, and thereby conclude failure before start due to their personal choices. Group two may be for beer. Then you have the general critics. I guess I won't even comment upon them except to say that they generally believe that their facts led them to an intelligent conclusion. What they don't consider to incorporate into their hypothesis theory base is that maybe they don't have enough information to make an intelligent decision about this. Having said that, the study of metaphysics can lead you to a vast amount of subjects and theories. One topic I had studied dealt with the spin rate in the molecular structure of water. So as I did my diet, I remembered that. The theory was that water that was not moving along a natural course was vibrating at a slower over all rate. So what I did was shook my bottled water. Now when it came to my beer reward system, I had to consider what I wanted the beer to do. I wanted the beer to cut or liquefy the fat in my system. So I decided the best way to enhance both features was to "chug" the beer. You see, once the bottle is turned upside down, the air

rushes to the bottom of the bottle. Holding my lips to the opening I would draw

the beer out rapidly. This action seemed to do two things. First, great amounts of

foam bubbles would be in the bottle. Second, the rapid drinking action would

seem to bloat my stomach. And so the concept of foam, bubbles, and internal

cleaning pressure. "Chug!" Now that's strange, I just thought of what will

happen if they start recommending a beer a day. Aaah, like they do about, Aaah,

WINE. I didn't hear anybody say "Wine O!"

IMAGES: THE CORE

< Front Cover Image From Back Pack Books: 1001 Facts About Ancient Egypt:

by Scott Steedman / Lower Image From Alcohol by Elaine Landau Page 10:

Corbis Images (Bettmann) >

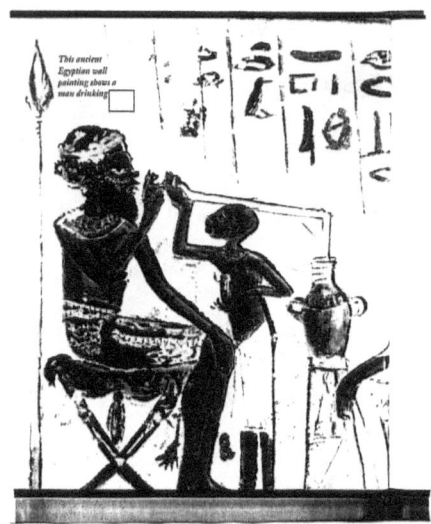

This ancient
Egyptian wall
painting shows a
man drinking

This is the core of the story about how I transformed myself from 283 plus pounds in mid May 2003, to 172 pounds on May 23, 2004. I explain what scientific data I found out about the human body. I also include the theories I combined to achieve my objective of losing 100 pounds. I feel that if I would have known years ago what I know today, I would have never suffered as I did. Now my objective is to try to help the people who are trying to help themselves improve their quality of life. I believe the clock of obesity can be turned backward. Best of luck, your friend Frank!

REAR COVER

I now realize that anyone can make something so simple into a complex problem. How does the body work? My research says simply: 1) either the human body is burning carbohydrates or protein for fuel, 2) extra carbohydrates eaten over those burned are stored as fat, and 3) when a person consumes very low or no carbohydrates they enter into a state of fat conversion burning called ketosis. A fat burning diet plan that induces ketosis is called a ketogenic diet. The missing link seems to be a lack of understanding that the human system can be maintained in one of three states: 1) plant eater which is called herbivore, 2) meat eater which is called carnivore, or 3) a mixture of both which is called omnivore. The final concern appears to be fluid consumption. My research model shows that when one eats only protein like the carnivores, one needs to consume larger amounts of water than in one of the other eating methods. Simply just look at the king of the jungle. The lion! I should also mention that my research found that Eskimos living above the Arctic Circle "eat virtually no carbohydrate and do fine." In addition I found a secret beverage high in water content that was as old as Egypt. This is how I lost 100 pounds using 20 pennies a day. After understanding the science all I needed to know was what I could eat? Just as they say, my body began to yo-yo. Then I began to search some more.

According to the scientific data I found, "in one hundred percent of obese people there is internal damage" to a specific organ. I have recently started to work upon that issue which I am going to write about later in another book. I did find the way to stabilize my weight and now eat as I want. This is knowledge that I hope can help you if you really want to help yourself. With all of my love, 168 pounds on February 24, 2006 Frank Jr. .

P. S. Tell somebody!!! Look for my other books on hermeneutics, kundalini, metaphysics, Egyptian ciphers, movie ciphers, Tai Chi, Karate, Tantra, and more on the web at lulu.com or unseenbooks.com. 3.14 out!

www.ingramcontent.com/pod-product-compliance
Lightning Source LLC
Chambersburg PA
CBHW031246280526
45784CB00004B/1744